Musculoskeletal X-rays

for Medical Students and Trainees

This title is also available as an e-book.
For more details, please see
www.wiley.com/buy/9781118458730
or scan this QR code:

Musculoskeletal X-rays

for Medical Students and Trainees

Andrew K. Brown
Consultant Rheumatologist
York Teaching Hospital NHS Trust; and
Senior Lecturer in Medical Education and Rheumatology
Hull York Medical School

David G. King
Consultant Musculoskeletal Radiologist
York Teaching Hospital NHS Trust; and
Honorary Senior Lecturer
Hull York Medical School

WILEY Blackwell

Library of Congress Cataloging-in-Publication Data

Names: Brown, Andrew K., author. | King, David G., author.
Title: Musculoskeletal X-rays for medical students and trainees / Andrew K. Brown, David G. King.
Description: Chichester, West Sussex, UK ; Malden, MA : John Wiley & Sons Inc., 2015. |
  Includes bibliographical references and index. | Description based on print version record and CIP data
  provided by publisher; resource not viewed.
Identifiers: LCCN 2014040930 (print) | LCCN 2014040575 (ebook) | ISBN 9781118458716 (Adobe PDF) |
  ISBN 9781118458723 (ePub) | ISBN 9781118458730 (pbk.)
Subjects: | MESH: Musculoskeletal Diseases–radiography.
Classification: LCC RC925.7 (print) | LCC RC925.7 (ebook) | NLM WE 141 | DDC 616.7/07572–dc23
LC record available at http://lccn.loc.gov/2014040930

A catalogue record for this book is available from the British Library.

Wiley also publishes its books in a variety of electronic formats. Some content that appears in print may not be available in electronic books.

Cover images: © Andrew K. Brown and David G. King

Set in 10/13pt Frutiger by SPi Global, Pondicherry, India

Printed and bound by CPI Group (UK) Ltd, Croydon, CR0 4YY

C9781118458730_220324

Contents

Preface

X-rays of bones and joints play a central role in musculoskeletal medicine and surgery, but the approach to evaluation and interpretation of X-rays is not always well taught or easily understood. This book should provide greater insight into the mysteries of the plain film X-ray and is ideal for medical students, doctors in training, physiotherapists, nurse practitioners and radiographers.

The book covers radiological anatomy as well as the main areas of pathology in which plain film assessment is clinically useful. The importance of correlation with relevant clinical findings and other imaging modalities will be highlighted and discussed where appropriate.

To make the radiological signs clear, each illustration consists of a pair of images, the first a standard X-ray and the second with coloured overlays added to precisely define each abnormality. By covering up the second image, the reader can also use this format to practise X-ray interpretation.

Our approach is largely based on the authors' combined experience of teaching medical students, trainees in emergency medicine, orthopaedics and rheumatology, as well as professions allied to medicine, over many years. By using this book, the reader will learn how the clues or signs found on an X-ray can be extracted and put together to aid in making a diagnosis and informing disease management.

We hope this book will provide an interesting and enjoyable way to obtain a clearer understanding of X-rays from the basics to more subtle findings across a broad range of musculoskeletal medicine.

Andrew K. Brown
David G. King

Acknowledgements

We would like to thank our colleagues at York Teaching Hospital for their help with finding suitable images for this book and especially Mike Pringle in the Department of Medical Illustration and Photography for his help and advice. We are also grateful to the students of Hull York Medical School for acting as subjects while we were developing our ideas and the material for this book.

PART 1
Introduction

1 Musculoskeletal X-rays

Introduction

Despite the availability of a wide range of imaging techniques to visualise musculoskeletal structures, plain radiographs or X-rays remain an important and widely used first-line investigation. It is probably the most readily available and least expensive imaging modality and is easily accessible to patients and healthcare professionals. As such, all medical professionals require at least a basic level of knowledge and training in the fundamental principles of requesting, interpreting and reporting plain radiographs of bones and joints.

Musculoskeletal X-rays for Medical Students and Trainees, First Edition. Andrew K. Brown and David G. King.
© 2017 John Wiley & Sons, Ltd. Published 2017 by John Wiley & Sons, Ltd.

Basic principles of requesting plain radiographs of bones and joints

Which structures?

Before requesting an X-ray, the clinician should already have a good idea of the likely nature of the clinical problem and which musculoskeletal structures may be affected and what may or may not be visualised on an X-ray. For example, radiographs are best at detecting pathological changes in bones, joints and cartilage, such as joint space narrowing, fracture, subluxation and dislocation. However, many soft tissue structures such as ligaments, tendons and synovium are not well visualised, and alternative imaging may be more appropriate to provide additional useful information to aid diagnosis and treatment.

Clinical assessment including the patient's symptoms and a physical examination will usually determine the site or region that is to be evaluated by X-ray. Exceptions may include a patient with rheumatoid arthritis where X-rays of both hands and feet may be used to evaluate the extent of disease or structural damage which may be repeated serially to compare any disease progression over time.

Which views?

It is important to consider which views are chosen to visualise a particular region of interest. This is because the X-ray beam creates a two dimensional shadow of a structure so selecting the correct view will maximise sensitivity. A basic principle is that two views should be requested, ideally 90° apart, which are usually obtained in antero-posterior (AP) and lateral or oblique views. This is particularly important in a trauma context where fracture or dislocation may be missed if only a single view is acquired but may be less important for the assessment of arthritis. There are a number of established techniques and protocols for optimal image acquisition using standardised views of most musculoskeletal sites. Specialist views may also be considered in particular clinical situations, such as a 'skyline view' for the patello-femoral joint or 'through-mouth view' for the cervical spine. As well as the particular plane used to acquire the radiographic image, the position of the patient should also be considered. For example, weight-bearing views with the patient in a standing position are often much more informative in evaluating cartilage loss in the knees of a patient with osteoarthritis or in providing additional information concerning biomechanical changes in the feet.

Compare both sides and review previous images

Particularly in equivocal cases, it may be informative to compare findings in a symptomatic area with the same region on the opposite side of the body or to look at the same region on a previous X-ray. For example, in a patient with hip pain, an AP X-ray of the pelvis allows some comparison between both hip joints, or in a patient with rheumatoid arthritis, comparison with a previous X-ray of the hands allows interpretation of any progression of erosive joint damage.

Correlation with clinical and other imaging findings

Any X-ray findings always need to be interpreted in clinical context, with an individual's symptoms, clinical examination findings and any other investigation results in mind. It may be necessary to perform additional imaging using alternative techniques such as ultrasound, computed tomography or magnetic resonance imaging, which may offer important additional or confirmatory information. Discussion with a specialist musculoskeletal radiologist is frequently helpful, and sharing and reviewing more challenging cases at a musculoskeletal radiology meeting involving clinicians and radiologists are often productive.

Safety considerations

Whilst undertaking a radiographic assessment is a well-regulated process and is generally considered safe, it is important to remember that the procedure exposes a patient to ionising radiation and a number of important safety precautions need to be considered. This is particularly important in children and young adults and when the area includes any organ which is more sensitive to ionising radiation such as the thyroid, breasts or gonads. In women of childbearing age if the area involves the abdomen, spine or pelvis, it is essential to ask the patient about the possibility of pregnancy and an X-ray in these circumstances should only be performed if absolutely necessary, such as a suspected pelvic fracture.

The amount of radiation exposure varies depending on the structure being visualised. Radiographs of deeper structures, such as the pelvis or lumbar spine, subject the patient to considerably greater radiation exposure than that of more peripheral structures, such as an examination of a single limb joint. The number of views and images obtained are proportional to the amount of radiation received. In all circumstances, it is important to be able to justify any radiation exposure on the basis of potential risk and benefit. The Department of Health Policy on Ionising Radiation (Medical Exposure) Regulations 2000 [1] covers these aspects in detail.

Basic principles of examining and reporting plain radiographs of bones and joints

Everyone should have a straightforward strategy for reviewing and interpreting musculoskeletal X-rays, including some basic principles and a systematic approach that can be routinely followed. It can often feel intimidating to review, interpret and describe an X-ray, but this need not be complex or jargon-heavy and confident use of simple descriptive language is all that is required. Undoubtedly, knowledge of musculoskeletal anatomy and understanding of pathological processes affecting bone, cartilage, joints and soft tissues will help, but a lot of information can be gained from describing any obvious abnormal or different appearances using simple descriptions, words and phrases. Even if you see an abnormality, it is still important to continue to evaluate the whole X-ray in case other findings are present. If an obvious change is not present or immediately apparent, then it is useful to be able to fall back on a standard framework with which to organise your thoughts and report your observations. An example of such an approach is outlined as follows:

1. *Check patient identification details and labelling.*
   Do the patient and X-ray identification details correspond, is it the correct X-ray being viewed, date and time, left or right?
2. *Is the image quality satisfactory? Are imaging angles optimal?*
   Consider densities, penetration and blackening of film (see "X-ray densities" below) and any inappropriate rotation and viewing angles. Also consider all additional views and patient position, has the region of interest been included?

X-ray densities

To understand the appearance of different densities on an X-ray, it is useful to consider the basic concept of how it has been produced. The image is essentially a shadow made by sending X-rays through an area of the body onto a detector behind. For about 100 years, the detector used was film. More recently, film has been swapped for electronic digital detectors but the concept remains the same. Where there is only air between the X-ray source and the detector, such as in the area around a limb, the film will be very exposed, that is blackened. Dense structures, such as bone, will stop most X-rays and the film will be less exposed, that is more white. Soft tissues produce intermediate shades of grey.

Assuming there is no metallic foreign body or other man-made artefact, there are only four densities to think about on an X-ray: calcium is white and gas is black. Of the soft tissues, fat is a darker shade of grey because it is a little less dense to X-rays than other soft tissues. All other soft tissues are the same lighter shade of grey, as is fluid (see Figure 1.1).

---

3. *Describe any obvious abnormality using simple descriptive language.*
   Name the specific bone (e.g. right tibia) and describe the location of any abnormality (e.g. proximal, middle or distal; head, neck or shaft; cortex or medulla). Basic terminology used for the paediatric and adult skeleton is shown in Figure 1.2. A combination of these terms and specific anatomical names should be used.
4. *Use a systematic approach to consider specific musculoskeletal structures (bones, joints, cartilage and soft tissues).*
   - Bone alignment – are there any changes in position which may suggest a fracture or dislocation?
   - Bone cortices – follow the outline of each bone as any breach in the cortex may indicate a fracture or an erosive arthritis.
   - Bone texture – Altered density or disruption in the usual trabecular pattern within the substance of the bone may indicate pathology.
   - Joint and cartilage – a careful look at the joint space may demonstrate changes such as joint space narrowing due to cartilage loss or calcification of the cartilage (chondrocalcinosis) or new bone formation (e.g. osteophytes in osteoarthritis).

- Soft tissues – remember to look at the soft tissues as well as the bones as they can hold helpful clues. For example, it may be possible to see if joint swelling is present and, therefore, that there must be something significant wrong with that joint. This will be discussed further in the chapter on trauma but also applies to any cause of joint swelling.

5. *Review all views and X-ray images, compare both sides and adjacent joints and re-examine any previous imaging.*

6. *Always consider clinical findings and correlation with other imaging and test results.*

7. *If there is still uncertainty, review all the available information once more, discuss the case with a musculoskeletal radiologist, and consider reviewing the case at a multidisciplinary radiology conference.*

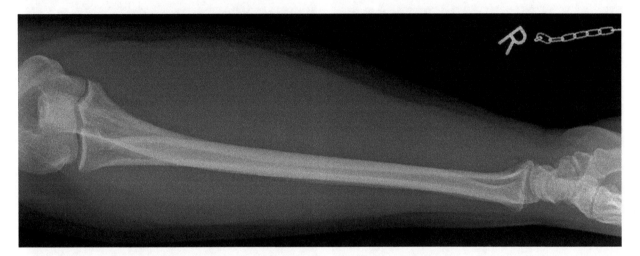

Figure 1.1 X-ray of the forearm illustrating the naturally occurring densities in a patient. White = calcium (in bone), dark grey = fat, lighter grey = all other soft tissue structures. Surrounding air is black.

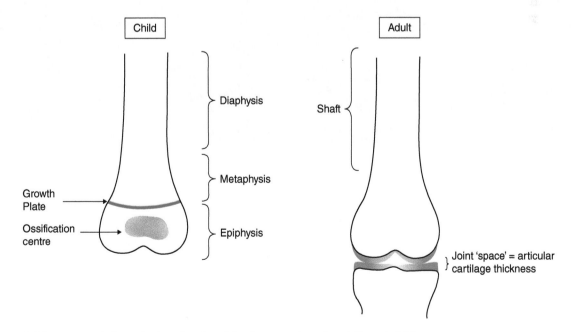

Figure 1.2 Recommended terminology for describing bone anatomy in adults and children.

Normal anatomy on musculoskeletal X-rays

This section features a series of paired standard X-ray images of each region, annotated with important anatomical structures. It will be useful to refer back to these as you read through the remaining chapters.

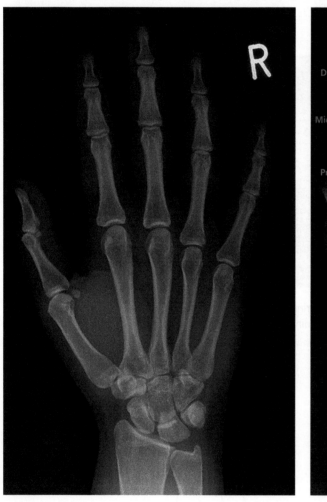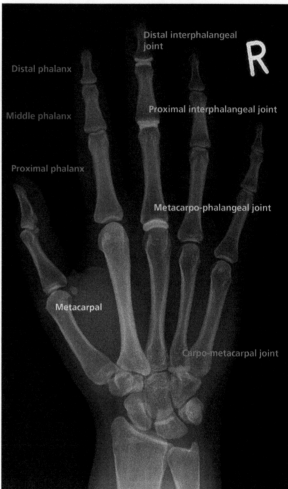

Figure 1.3 Normal hand.

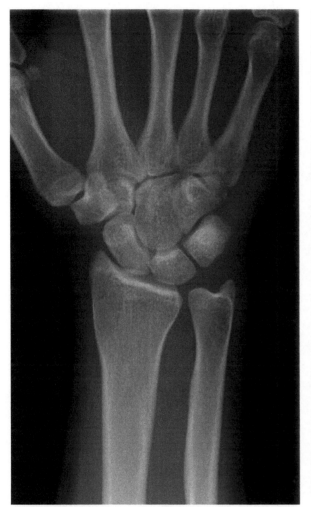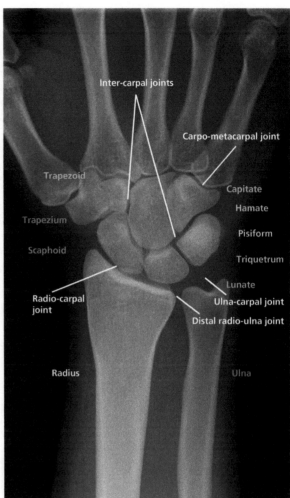

Figure 1.4 Normal wrist, PA view.

Remember trapez*ium* is adjacent to the th*um*b.

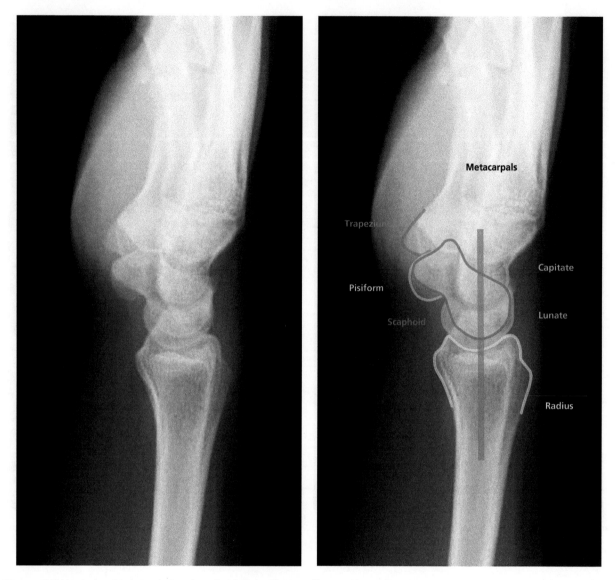

Figure 1.5 Normal wrist, lateral view (see the 4 Cs in Chapter 2).

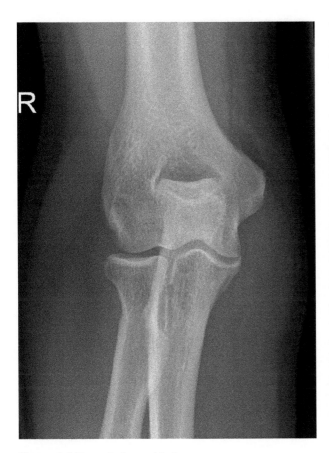
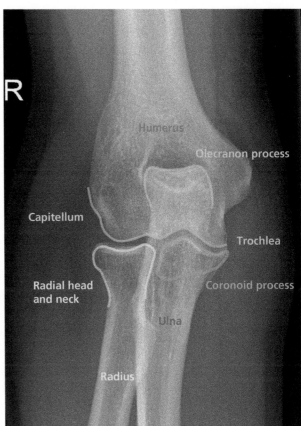

Figure 1.6 Normal elbow, AP view.

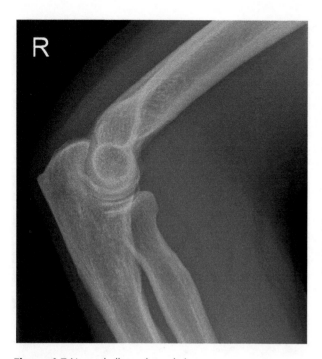
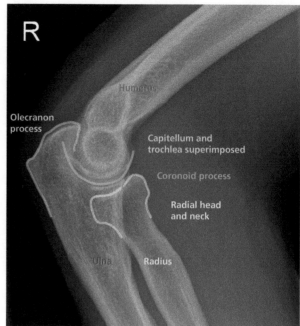

Figure 1.7 Normal elbow, lateral view.

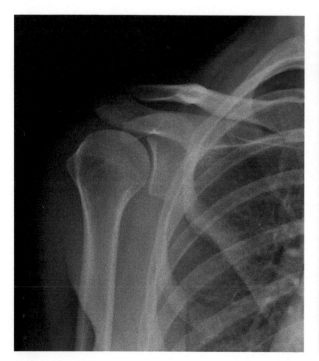
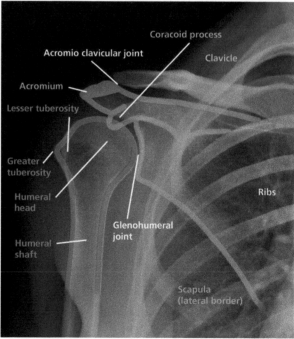

Figure 1.8 Normal shoulder, AP view.

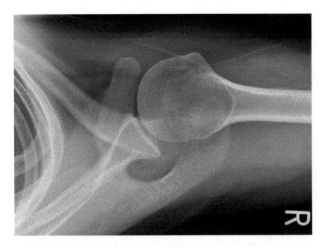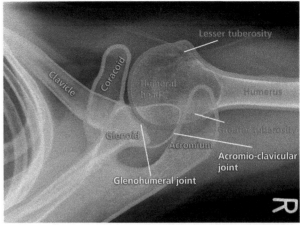

Figure 1.9 Normal shoulder, axial view.

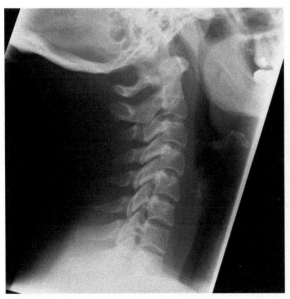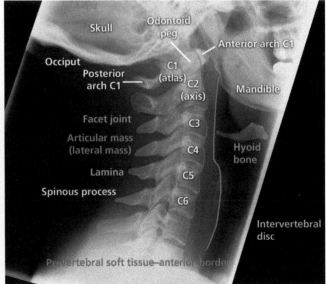

Figure 1.10 Normal cervical spine, lateral view.

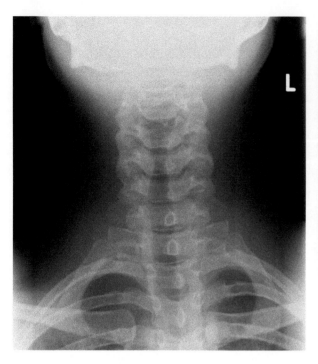
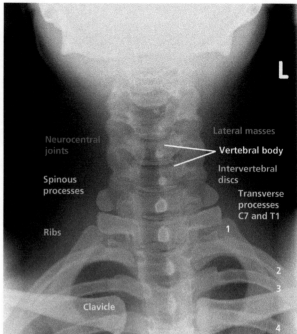

Figure 1.11 Normal cervical spine, AP view.

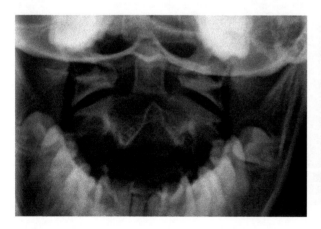
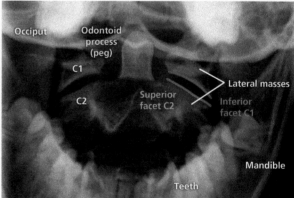

Figure 1.12 Normal cervical spine, through-mouth view.

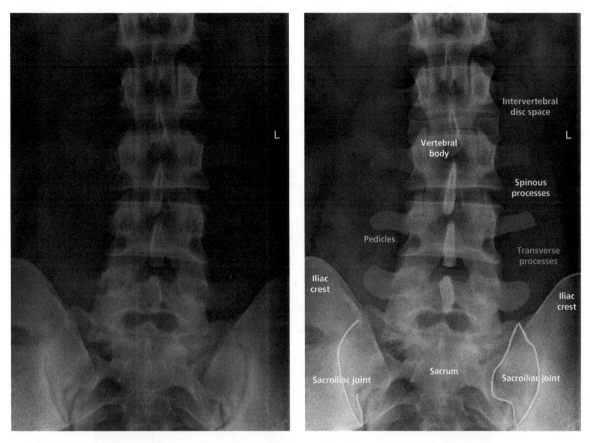

Figure 1.13 Normal lumbar spine and sacroiliac joints, AP view.

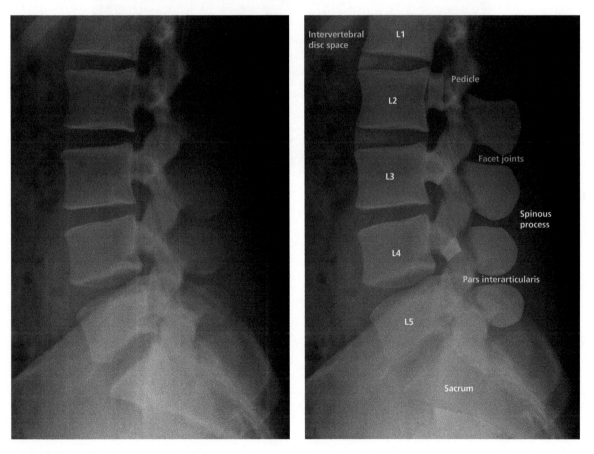

Figure 1.14 Normal lumbar spine, lateral view.

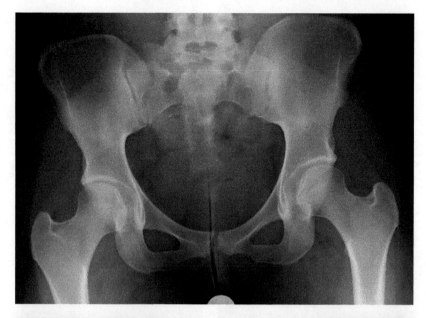

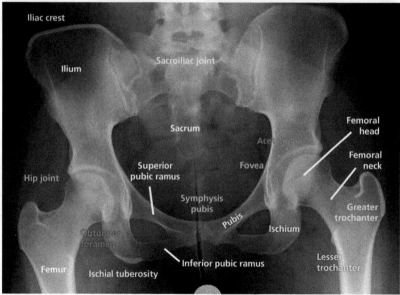

Figure 1.15 Normal pelvis, AP view.

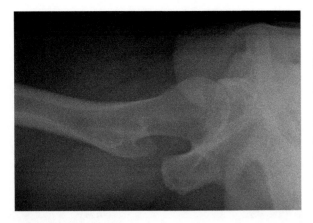
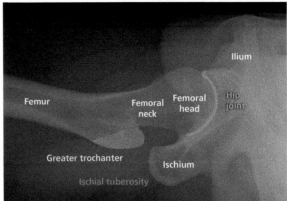

Figure 1.16 Normal hip, lateral view.

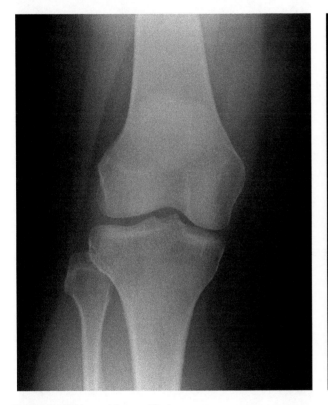
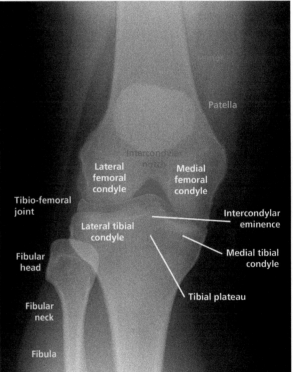

Figure 1.17 Normal knee, AP view.

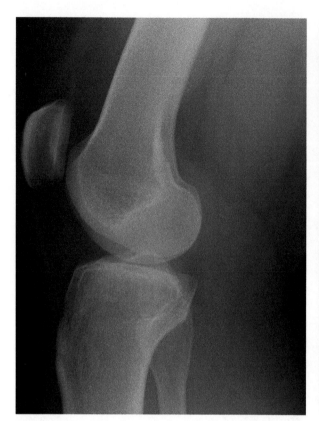 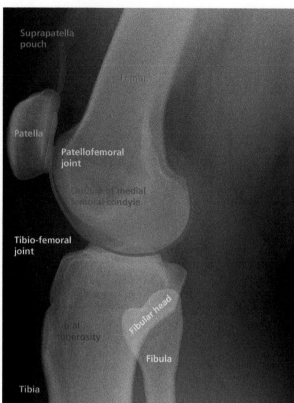

Figure 1.18 Normal knee, lateral view.

On the lateral view, the medial condyle is round; lateral femoral condyle is indented due to a sulcus.

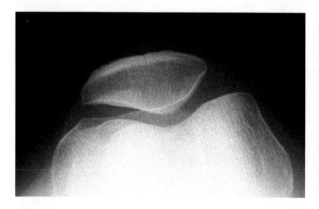 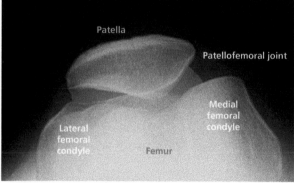

Figure 1.19 Normal knee, sky-line patella view.

*On the patella, the **L**ateral patellar facet = **L**arge*

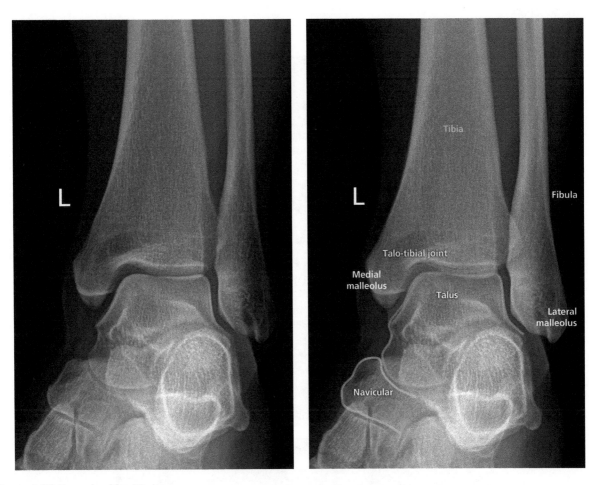

Figure 1.20 Normal ankle, AP view.

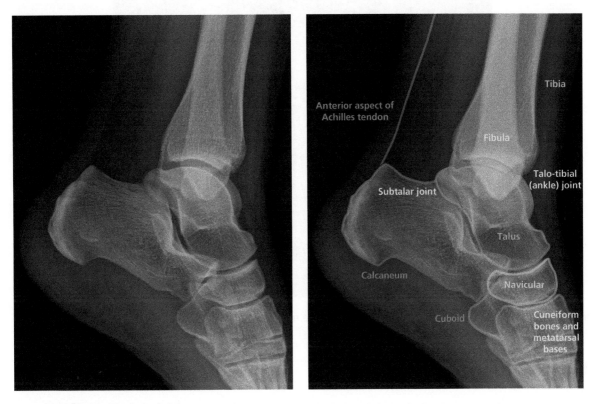

Figure 1.21 Normal ankle, lateral view.

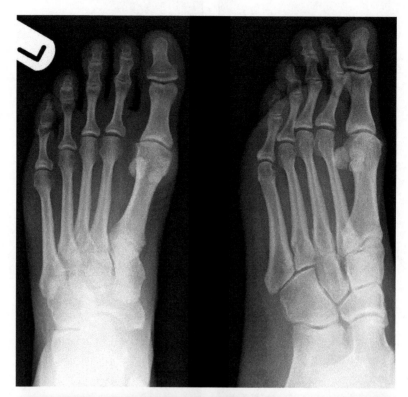

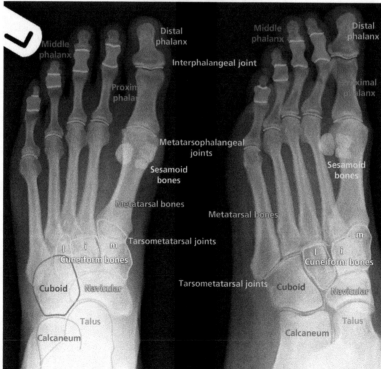

Figure 1.22 Normal foot, AP and oblique views (note bipartite medial sesamoid bone which is a normal variant). Cuneiform bones: l = lateral, i = intermediate, m = medial.

Reference

1. The Ionising Radiation (Medical Exposure) Regulations 2000 (IR(ME)R 2000), The Department of Health 2012. Available at: https://www.gov.uk/government/publications/the-ionising-radiation-medical-exposure-regulations-2000 (accessed on 19 September 2014).

PART 2
Pathology

2 Trauma

Bone and joint injuries

Introduction
This section describes general concepts of trauma imaging, including how to evaluate an X-ray in order to detect bone and joint injuries and how to describe the findings. Basic X-ray signs and more subtle clues for spotting injuries are also described. Some specific injuries are discussed in the second part of the chapter, including a section on paediatric injuries. Other imaging modalities, such as MRI, CT and ultrasound, have an important role in trauma, and so are mentioned when relevant.

X-ray appearances of fractures
In most cases, a fracture is visible because there is a radiolucent (dark) line running through the bone. The bony fragments on either side of the fracture separate, leaving a less dense gap between them. This is often accompanied by some change in the normal alignment at the fracture site (displacement) (Figure 2.1). When a fracture is undisplaced, the line of the fracture may be less easy to see (Figure 2.2).

If the fragments are not separated or separation is obscured by the projection of the X-ray, the only sign of a fracture might be a subtle step or irregularity of the bony cortex (Figure 2.3). The cortex normally has a smooth contour, and it is important to follow this closely around the margin of each bone looking for any step or discontinuity.

If the bone fragments are impacted rather than separated, the fracture may show as a band of *increased* density. This is because the amount of bone per unit volume is doubled at the site where the two fragments have been forced into each other (Figure 2.4). A similar increase in density will also occur where fragments are overlapping due to the projection, rather than impacted.

Also, localised swelling of the soft tissues may be visible on the X-ray, adjacent to a recent injury. The skin contour over the fracture site is displaced by the swelling (Figure 2.5). Swelling

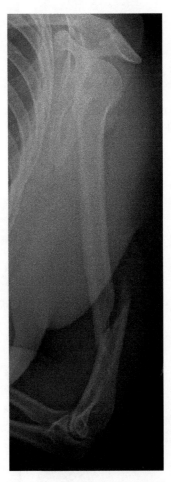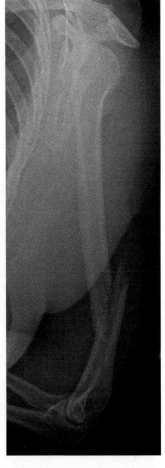

Figure 2.1 Fracture of the distal humerus. Signs: Deformity of the bone due to displacement at the fracture site. The darker fracture line (orange) interrupts the dense bone structure.

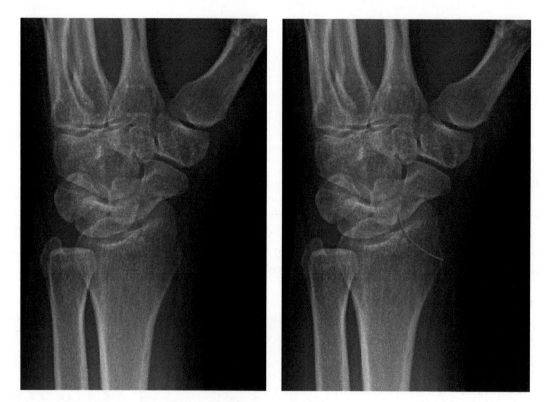

Figure 2.2 Undisplaced fracture of the radial styloid process. Signs: The normal shape of the bone is preserved, but a subtle less dense, that is dark, fracture line (orange) can be seen separating the radial styloid from the rest of the bone.

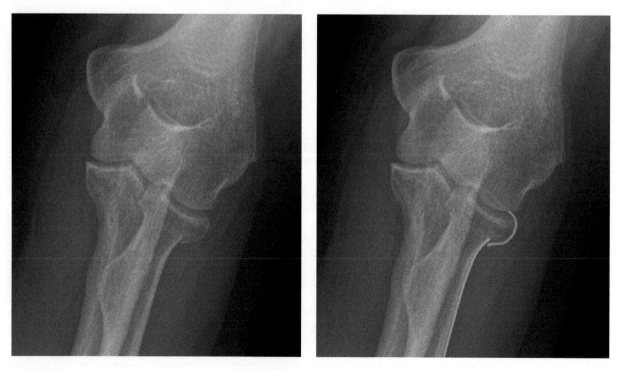

Figure 2.3 Minimally displaced fracture of the radial neck. Signs: The cortex normally has a smooth contour. Carefully following the cortex around the margin of the radius (yellow) reveals a small step just distal to the head.

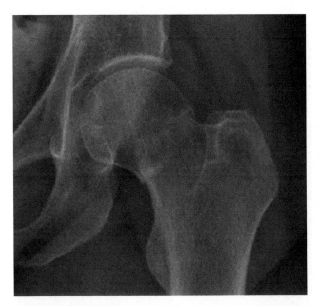
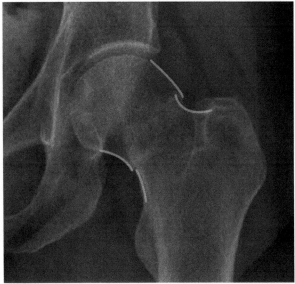

Figure 2.4 Minimally displaced fracture of the neck of the femur. Signs: Increased density partially crossing the femoral neck due to impaction at the fracture site (orange) and steps in the cortex medially and laterally (yellow).

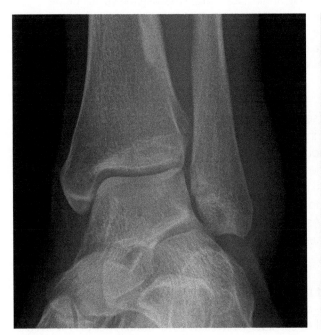
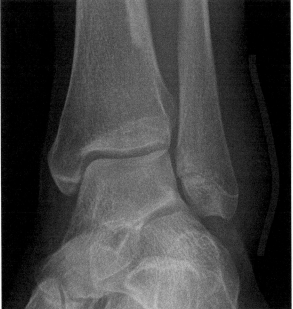

Figure 2.5 Soft tissue swelling overlying an undisplaced transverse fracture of the lateral malleolus (orange). The localised swelling is best appreciated by looking at the silhouette of the skin surface against the darker surrounding air (green).

of the soft tissues can occur in the absence of a fracture and therefore it is a secondary sign; nonetheless, it can be a useful clue pointing to an abnormality at the corresponding site.

Osteochondral fractures

The term 'osteochondral fracture' is used when there is a fracture of part of a joint surface. The injury involves an area of articular cartilage and the attached underlying bone. These injuries are caused when bone on one side of a joint impacts against the opposite side. When any injury involves a joint, it is important to look closely at the articular surfaces as osteochondral fractures are often subtle. Cartilage is not visible on X-rays, but the

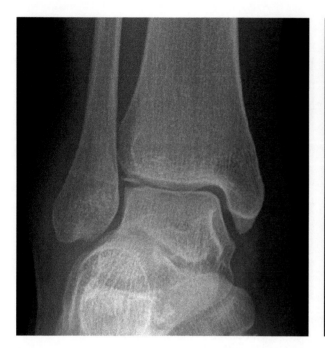
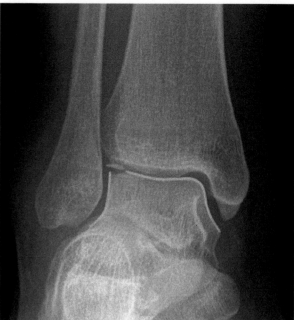

Figure 2.6 Osteochondral fracture of the lateral corner of the dome of the talus. Signs: Following the outline of the articular surface reveals an interruption in the cortex (yellow) and a small fragment of calcium density (green). This is slightly displaced and projected within the joint space. Fractures of the medial or lateral corner of the dome of the talus are relatively common but easy to miss on X-rays. In fact, one-third of fractures are not visible on initial X-rays. It is important to look closely at the dome of the talus in any patient with an ankle injury.

attached piece of bone from the articular cortex can be seen, often visible as a thin flake (Figure 2.6). It may be undisplaced or lie away from the 'donor' site elsewhere in the joint. For example, in the knee it may come to rest in the medial or lateral recess of the suprapatellar pouch. The bony component of the osteochondral fragment has a smooth, rounded articular surface on one side and an irregular uncorticated appearance on the surface which has fractured. Make a careful search for (i) any displaced intra-articular fragment and (ii) a defect in the articular cortex of the joint. Although the visible bony part of the fragment often appears small, there will be a larger attached articular cartilage component. As damage to a joint surface has long-lasting sequelae in terms of pain and stiffness, an apparently small fragment may have considerable significance.

Avulsion fractures
If a soft tissue structure is put under sufficient tension, it may either rupture or pull off a fragment from its bony attachment, that is an avulsion fracture. Therefore, avulsion fractures only occur at the insertions of ligaments, tendons, muscles or joint capsule. It is helpful to consider which soft tissue attachment is involved when looking at the X-ray (Figure 2.7).

Stress and insufficiency fractures
Although most fractures are caused by a single traumatic incident, a stress fracture can occur when a lesser degree of force is applied repeatedly. For example, stress fractures may be seen in the tibial shaft in sports which involve running; the pars interarticularis of the lumbar spine in fast bowlers; and the third metatarsal in people who undertake an unaccustomed amount of walking (Figure 2.8).

Stress fractures occur when repeated forces on the skeleton are abnormally high although the underlying bone strength is normal. However, if the skeleton is subjected to a normally tolerable force but the bone strength is low and a fracture occurs, this is known as an insufficiency fracture or a fragility fracture (Figure 2.9). This situation is most commonly seen in patients with osteoporosis.

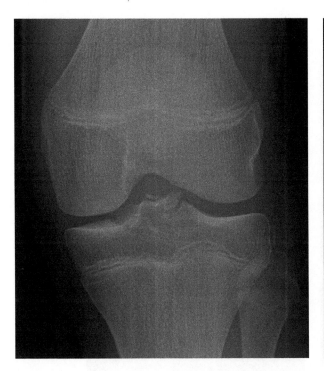
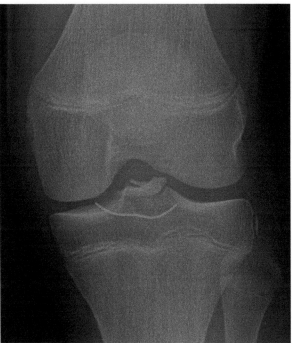

Figure 2.7 Two avulsion fractures are visible on the AP view of this adolescent patient's knee. The fragment coloured green is a fracture of the tibial eminence, avulsed by the anterior cruciate ligament. The fragment coloured orange is an avulsion of the tibial cortex by the attachment of the lateral joint capsule. Although this lateral injury looks innocuous, it has a strong association with ACL and meniscal tears and is named a Segond fracture.

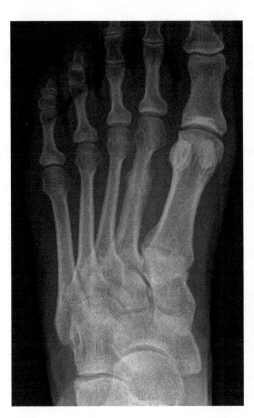
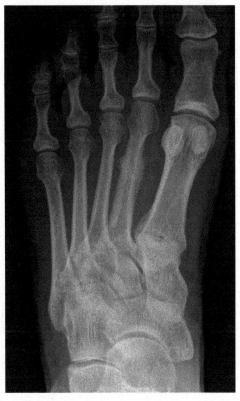

Figure 2.8 A typical stress fracture of the distal shaft of the index metatarsal. The fracture is undisplaced and no fracture line is visible on the film, but its presence is shown by the callus which has developed on either side of the fracture site (orange).

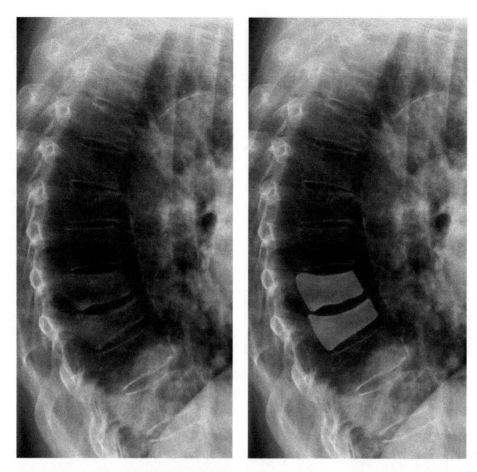

Figure 2.9 An elderly woman with back pain but no history of a specific injury. The film shows mildly and moderately severe wedge fractures of two vertebral bodies (blue). The fractures do not show specific radiological signs to indicate that they are fragility fractures. This comes from the history and exclusion of other causes.

Pathological fractures

The term 'pathological fracture' is generally used to describe a fracture caused by a focal lesion which has weakened the structure of the bone. A common cause is destructive bony metastatic disease (Figure 2.10), but pathological fractures also occur in association with benign lesions which weaken the bone structure.

What is not a fracture

There are a number of things which appear on X-rays which might resemble a fracture but are not, so it is useful to be aware of some of the more common pitfalls.

Accessory ossicles are a common normal variant. Characteristically they are small, rounded and lie adjacent to joints. They differ from fracture fragments in that they have a smooth surrounding cortex which covers all sides, whereas on a fracture fragment it is usually possible to find an area where the margin has a sharp, rather irregular appearance and lacks an overlying cortex which corresponds to where it was previously attached to its site of origin (Figure 2.11).

A skin crease projected over a bone may be visible on X-ray as a black line, similar to a fracture. However, following the line along its whole length will usually show that it extends beyond the margins of the bone, which could not be the case with a fracture (Figure 2.12).

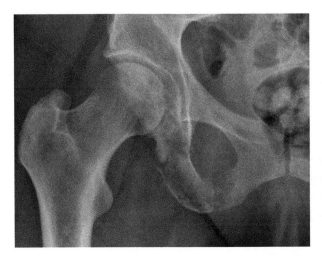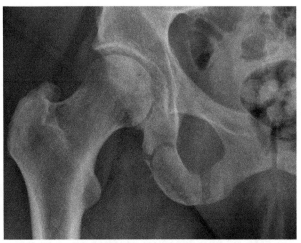

Figure 2.10 A pathological fracture of the right ischiopubic ramus. There are two fracture lines (orange) across the bone, but the underlying bone texture is also abnormal, with ill-defined lucency extending from the acetabulum to the inferior pubic ramus, due to the presence of a lytic metastasis (green). Compare the bone texture in this area with the normal appearance in the rest of the image.

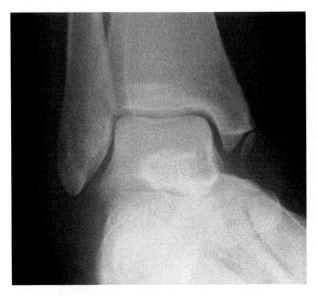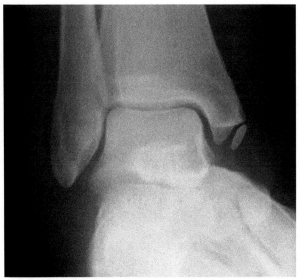

Figure 2.11 An accessory ossicle (blue) lying adjacent to the medial malleolus. Note that the ossicle is smooth and rounded and has a complete surrounding cortex.

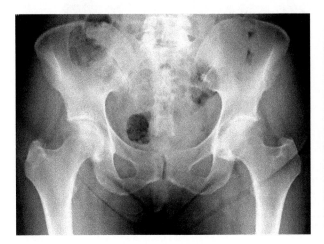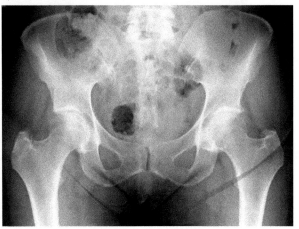

Figure 2.12 A soft tissue crease causing a dark line (blue) across the intertrochanteric region of the left femoral neck. Initially, this might be mistaken for a fracture, but the line can be followed into the soft tissues beyond the margins of the bone.

Describing fractures

To communicate a clear picture of a bony injury to a colleague, it helps to have a mental list of the relevant features which need to be evaluated and described:

Which bone has fractured?

Name the bone and include whether this is on the right or left side of the patient.

A letter 'R' or 'L' should always appear in the periphery of an X-ray to indicate the right or left side of the patient. For example, Figure 2.13 shows *a fracture of the right middle finger metacarpal*. (*Note*: In this book, the side markers are mostly cropped off the original images for reasons of space.)

The site of the fracture within that bone

In Figure 2.13, the fracture involves the *proximal shaft* of the metacarpal.

It is also important to note whether the fracture involves the articular surface of the bone. Any loss of the normal smooth articular surface may result in secondary osteoarthritis, and therefore these fractures may require different treatment to ensure very accurate reduction (Figure 2.14).

The number of fragments

Is it a simple two-part fracture or is it comminuted? When multiple fragments are present, the term comminuted or multi-fragmentary is used (Figure 2.15).

The orientation of the fracture

The metacarpal fracture shown in Figure 2.13 is transverse. The orientation of a fracture can also be longitudinal, oblique or, when a twisting force has occurred, spiral (Figure 2.16a–c).

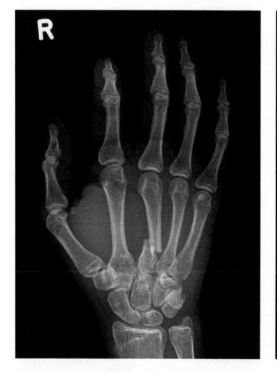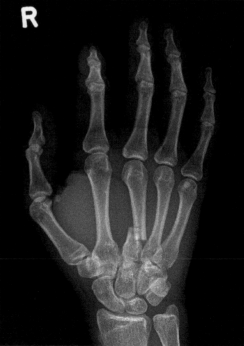

Figure 2.13 Fracture *site*: There is a fracture of the proximal shaft of the middle metacarpal of the right hand (orange).

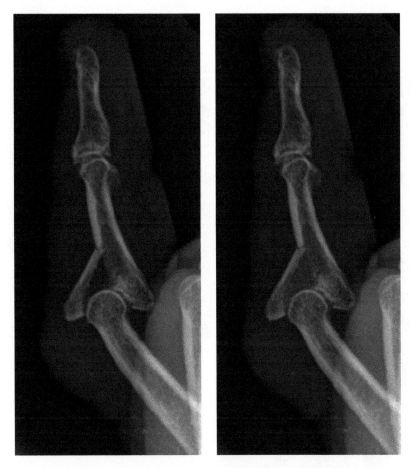

Figure 2.14 Articular surface involvement: This middle phalanx fracture extends into the proximal interphalangeal joint.

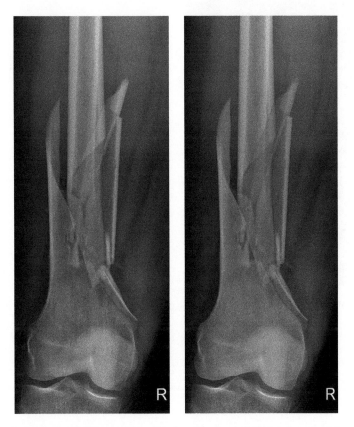

Figure 2.15 There are more than two bone fragments in this distal femoral shaft fracture, and therefore it is described as comminuted or multi-fragmentary.

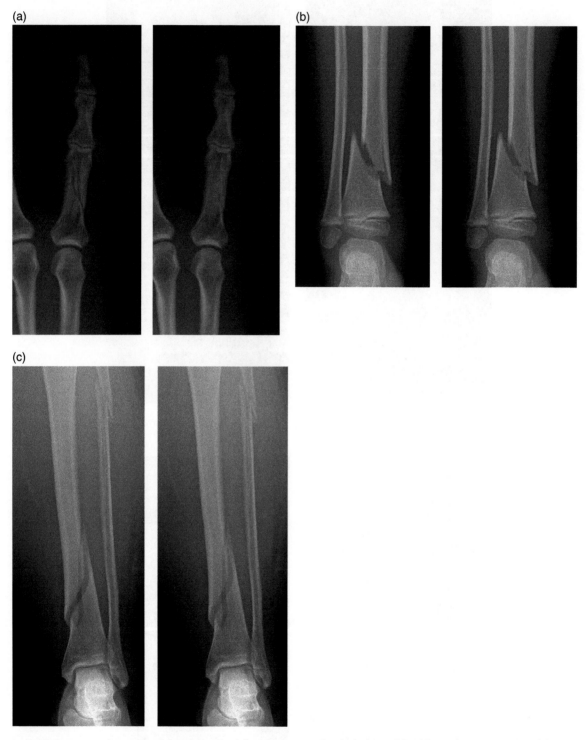

Figure 2.16 Fracture orientation: (a) Longitudinal fractures – proximal phalanx. (b) Oblique fracture – tibia. (c) Spiral fracture – tibia.

Displacement

When describing displacement, the position of the fragment distal to the fracture site is always described. Determine how the alignment of this fragment has changed from where it was before the injury, that is how has it moved away from the normal anatomical alignment. The 'anatomical position' (Figure 2.17) is the standard starting point from which any displacement is described.

Displacement can take the form of angulation, shift or a combination of these. Angulation and shift can both occur laterally, medially, anteriorly or posteriorly. There may also be proximal or distal shift. It is essential to look at two X-ray views at 90° to one another to appreciate displacement properly as it may be hidden on a single projection (Figure 2.18a and b). See example in Figure 2.19.

Similarly with dislocations, the position of the more distal of the bones forming the joint is stated and the bone proximal to the injury is used as the reference point (Figure 2.20).

In the case of dislocations, the name of the distal bone is often omitted. For example at the shoulder there may be an "anterior dislocation" or a "posterior dislocation" based on the position of the humeral head.

The term dislocation refers to a joint injury in which the two articular surfaces are no longer in contact, whereas in the case of subluxation there is contact between some part of the joint surfaces but the alignment is abnormal.

Rotational deformity cannot be accurately shown by X-rays and should be assessed clinically. Also when describing a fracture it is important to note if a fracture is open or closed, but again this is part of the clinical, rather than radiological, assessment.

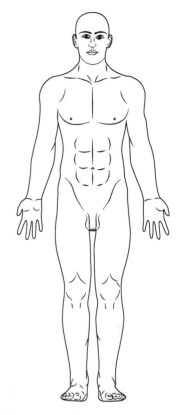

Figure 2.17 The anatomical position.

(a) (b)

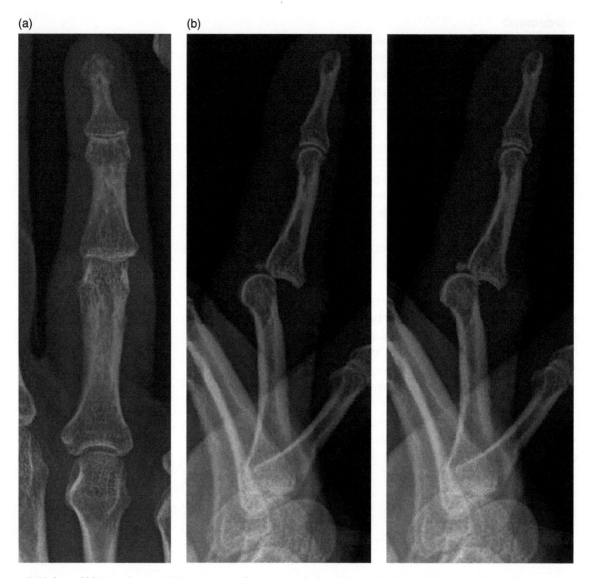

Figure 2.18 (a and b) Two views at 90° to one another are needed to detect injuries and also to evaluate displacement. This proximal interphalangeal joint injury is difficult to appreciate on the AP view, but the lateral film clearly demonstrates dorsal subluxation, with loss of congruity of the articular surfaces (blue). It also reveals the presence of a small fracture fragment (orange).

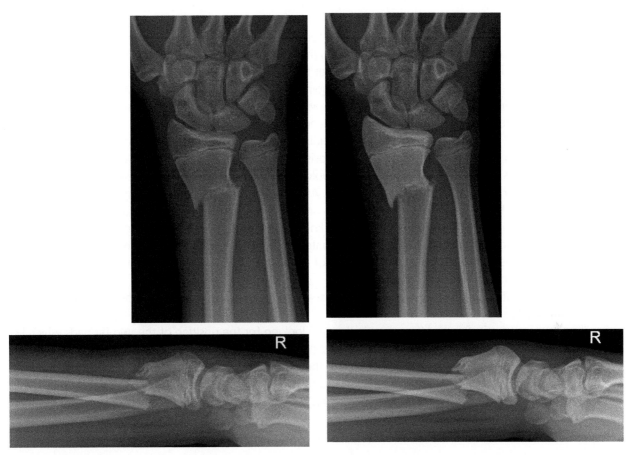

Figure 2.19 A fracture of the distal diaphysis of the radius. Evaluating the films for displacement of the distal fragment, the lateral view shows dorsal shift and the 'AP' view shows lateral shift and lateral angulation.

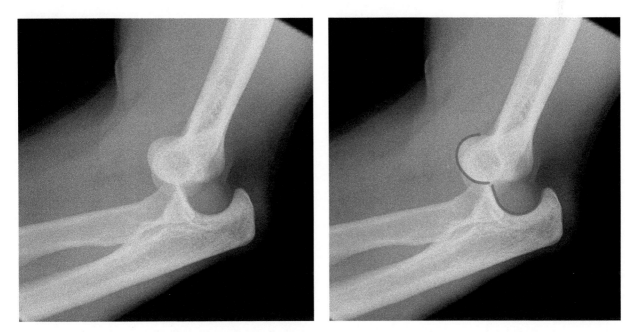

Figure 2.20 Dislocation of the elbow. Predominantly, the distal bones of the joint (radius and ulna) have moved posteriorly from their normal anatomical position. Articular surfaces of the trochlea and olecranon are in blue. The injury could be described thus: 'The radius and ulna have dislocated in a posterior direction', but this is usually shortened to, 'There is a posterior dislocation of the elbow'.

Other X-ray signs of joint injury

At certain joints, intra-articular swelling can be looked for using the lateral X-ray. Although swelling is not a specific sign, when present it does imply that there is significant pathology affecting that joint.

It is possible to tell if the knee is swollen by looking at the suprapatellar pouch on the lateral image. The suprapatellar pouch is a continuation of the knee joint which extends proximally between the femur and the quadriceps tendon. It can be seen on the lateral view, as a layer of lighter grey, because it is silhouetted on the anterior and posterior aspects by darker grey fat planes. In the normal situation, it is a thin structure with a thickness of around 2 mm (Figure 2.21). But when the joint is swollen, this thickness increases (Figure 2.22). The cause of swelling can be an effusion, a haemarthrosis or synovial thickening, and these will all have the same, light grey, density. If there is a fracture which involves one of the joint surfaces, bleeding from the fracture site will enter the joint and cause it to distend. At the same time, fat from the bone marrow may also pass through the fracture into the joint, where it floats on top of the blood as a separate layer. If there is sufficient fat present this 'lipohaemarthrosis', as it is known, can be detected on a horizontal-beam lateral X-ray because the two layers of fluid within the suprapatellar pouch have different densities (Figure 2.23).

A lipohaemarthrosis can be seen in about one-third of cases of intra-articular fracture of the knee, the other two-thirds having a simple haemarthrosis.

On a lateral view of the ankle, it may be possible to see swelling extending anteriorly from the joint (Figure 2.24a and b).

Swelling at the elbow is slightly different in that we are looking for the position of the two fat pads which lie inside the joint, rather than the fat planes outside. At the anterior and posterior aspects of the distal humerus, there are small fat pads which are normally situated in the olecranon and coronoid fossae, respectively. When there is increased fluid inside the joint, it gets underneath the fat pads and lifts them out of the fossae so they become conspicuous on a lateral X-ray (Figure 2.25a and b).

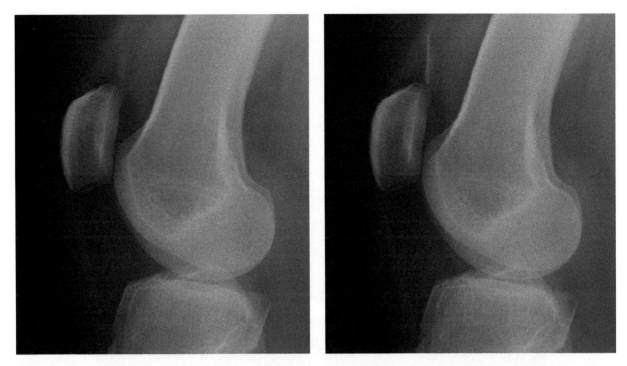

Figure 2.21 Normal lateral knee. The lighter grey suprapatellar pouch lies between the dark grey of the fat planes on its anterior and posterior aspects, and therefore its thickness can be seen. Normally, the thickness is just 2 or 3 mm (green).

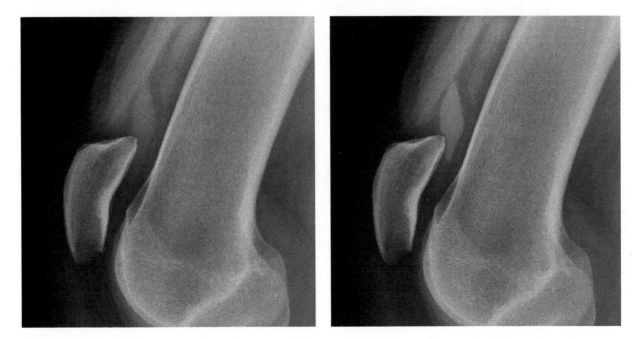

Figure 2.22 When the knee joint is swollen, the suprapatellar pouch can be seen to increase in thickness (green).

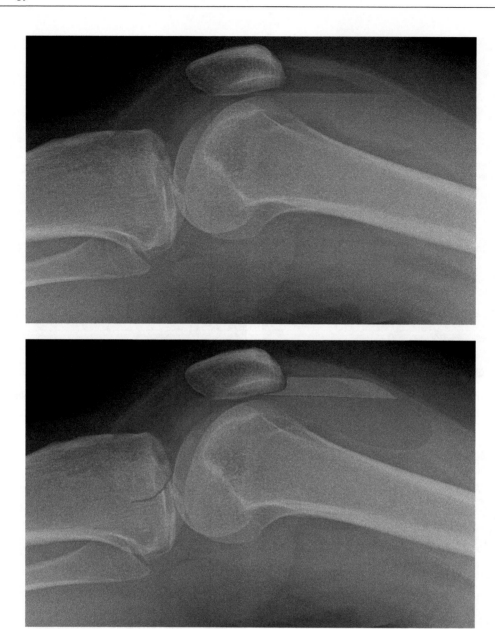

Figure 2.23 Lipohaemarthrosis in a patient with a fracture of the tibial joint surface. Low-density fat (yellow) forms a layer floating on top of denser blood (red) inside the suprapatellar pouch. Therefore, an intra-articular fracture must be present. A subtle fracture line is visible extending into the tibial joint surface (blue).

(a)

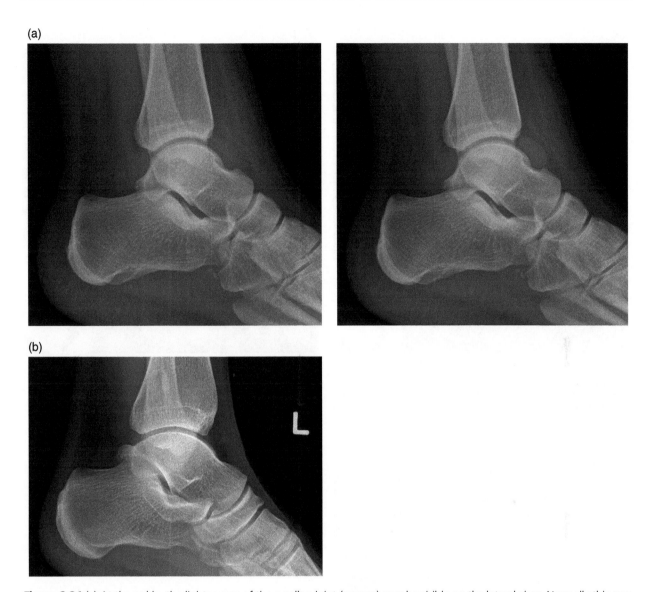

(b)

Figure 2.24 (a) At the ankle, the lighter grey of the swollen joint (orange) may be visible on the lateral view. Normally this area is occupied by a darker grey fat plane as in figure (b) for comparison.

(a)

(b)

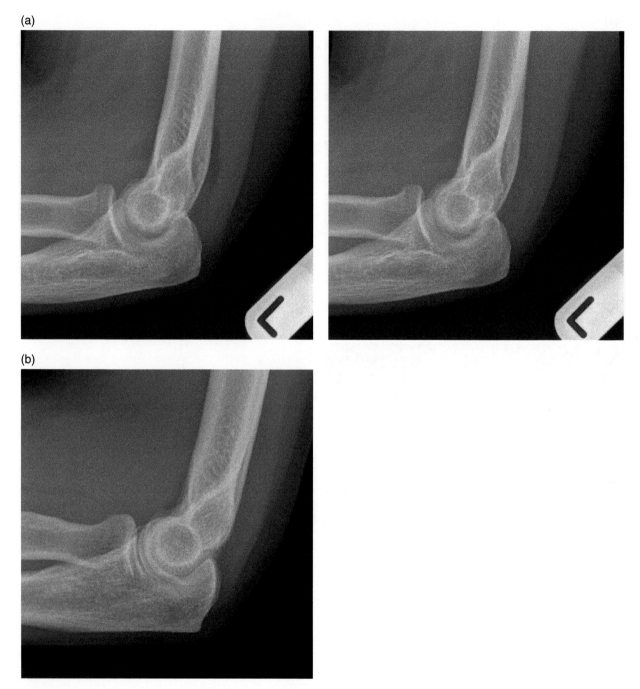

Figure 2.25 (a and b) Detecting swelling at the elbow also relies on contrast between fat and other tissues, but in a slightly different way. Here the anterior and posterior fat pads do not outline the joint capsule, but they can indicate the presence of joint swelling. They normally sit in the fossae on the anterior and posterior aspects of the distal humerus where they are barely visible on a lateral X-ray. However, increased joint fluid or synovial thickening gets underneath them in the fossae, lifting them out and pushing them superiorly so that they become more prominent (purple). Image (b) is normal for comparison.

Specific injuries

Many fractures and dislocations are relatively straightforward to diagnose on plain X-rays, but at certain sites it is useful to know which specific features to look for to get maximum information from the images and avoid common misses.

Shoulder

Because there is little bony confinement of the humeral head within the glenoid, this joint has a uniquely multidirectional and wide range of movement. However, this comes at the cost of reduced intrinsic stability, and consequently the shoulder dislocates more frequently than any other joint.

When X-rays are performed after trauma, the antero-posterior (AP) view is standard. The second view at 90° to this may be axial (as if looking from either above or below) or lateral (as if looking from the side). In evaluating shoulder dislocations and other injuries, understanding the radiological anatomy is important, so you may wish to refer back to Figures 1.8 and 1.9. By identifying the glenoid and the humeral head on both views, it is possible to check if the head is sitting centrally in the glenoid. If this is not the case, it is dislocated or subluxed. Ninety-five per cent of shoulder dislocations are anterior (Figure 2.26a). On the AP image, it can be seen that the articular surface of the humeral head no longer has a normal alignment with the glenoid, but it is not possible to see if the head lies in front of or behind the glenoid without a second view taken perpendicular to the first. This can be axial (Figure 2.26b) or lateral (Figure 2.26c) projection. On either of these, check which aspect of the scapula is anterior and which is posterior. One way to do this is by identifying the coracoid process, which resembles a bony finger pointing forwards. Once you can orientate yourself and also identify the glenoid, you should be able to see (i) the articular surface of the humerus no longer sits neatly in the glenoid, with their articular surfaces parallel to one another, and (ii) if the humeral dislocation is anterior or posterior. Five per cent of shoulder dislocations are posterior (Figure 2.27a and b). Posterior shoulder dislocation is an injury which is commonly associated with a seizure or an electric shock.

Dislocation of any joint may be accompanied by fractures, so always make a careful search for any separate bony fragments and other signs of fracture on both the initial X-ray and also the post-reduction views (Figure 2.28).

Elbow

Elbow fractures, for example of the radial head or neck, are often subtle and the fat pad sign discussed earlier might be an important clue to the presence of a significant injury (Figure 2.29a and b).

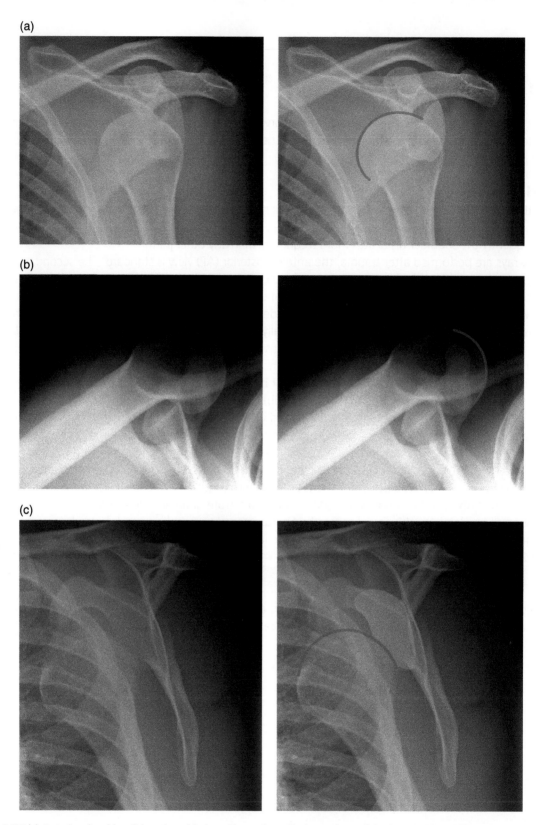

Figure 2.26 (a) Anterior shoulder dislocation, AP view. Signs: The articular surface of the humeral head (green) no longer lies congruently against that of the glenoid (yellow). The head is displaced medially and is projected over the glenoid. (b) Anterior shoulder dislocation, axial view. By identifying the bony anatomy, it is possible to find the articular surfaces of the humeral head and glenoid and again see that they are not articulating with one another. Also by determining the anterior aspect of the scapula, for example by identifying the coracoid process (purple), it is possible to say that the humerus has dislocated anteriorly. (c) Anterior shoulder dislocation, lateral view. As with the previous projection, the humeral head, glenoid and anterior and posterior aspects of the scapula should be checked to establish that there is an anterior dislocation of the shoulder.

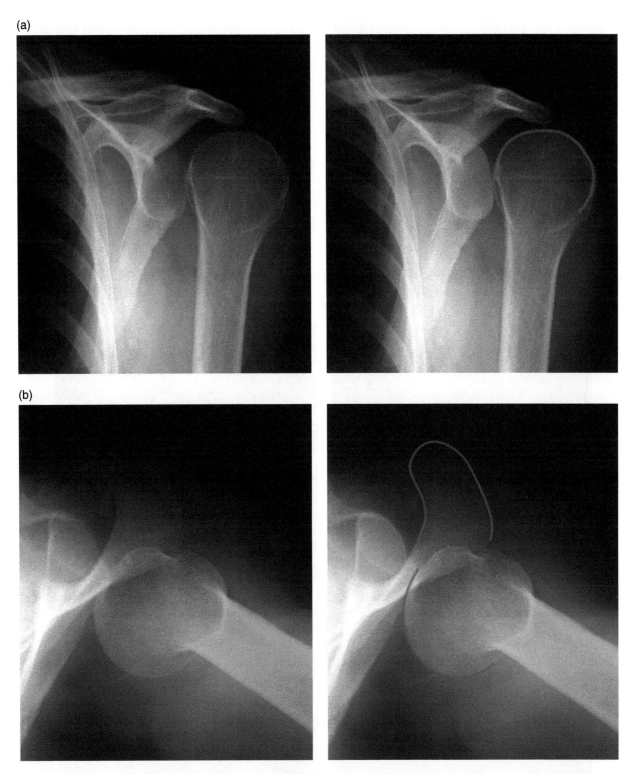

Figure 2.27 (a) Posterior shoulder dislocation. Signs: On this AP view, the dislocation is not obvious because the humeral head (green) lies level with the articular surface of the glenoid (yellow). However, an abnormal amount of the surface of the glenoid is visible – the 'bare glenoid' sign. The humerus has a 'light bulb' appearance caused by internal rotation. The arm is locked in internal rotation in patients who have a posterior dislocation. (b) Posterior shoulder dislocation, axial view. Less of the scapula is visible on this film as the patient has had difficulty abducting the shoulder for the X-ray. As a result, the corocoid process is not included on the film, but once again identification of the bony anatomy allows the dislocation and the fact that it is posterior to be confirmed. The acromion (orange) can be seen turning anteriorly to meet the lateral end of the clavicle at the acromioclavicular joint.

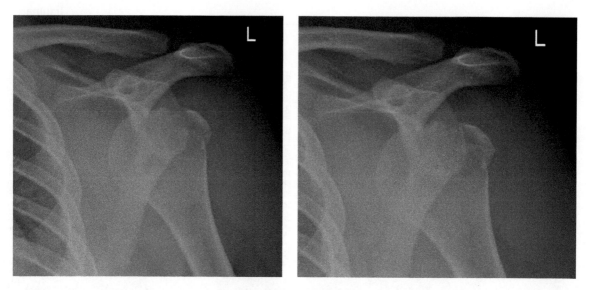

Figure 2.28 Fracture of the greater tuberosity of the humerus with shoulder dislocation. Signs: Fracture lines (orange) causing breaks in the cortex and running through the bone between the greater tuberosity and the humeral head.

(a)

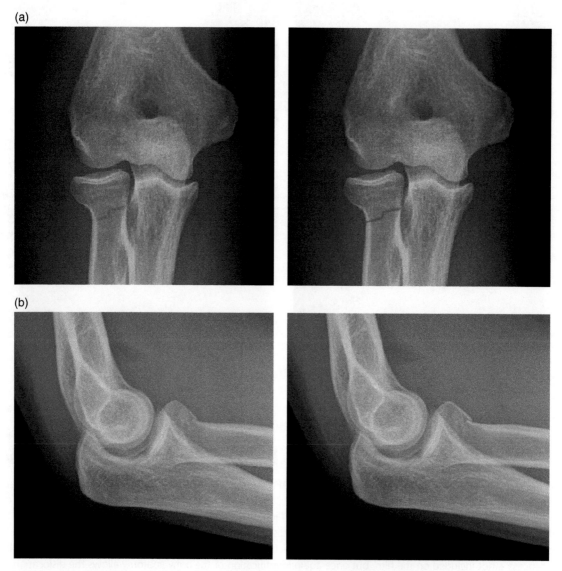

(b)

Figure 2.29 (a and b) The elevated anterior fat pad (orange) is a clue that there is a significant abnormality. The neck of the radius shows a subtle break in the cortex (yellow) and slight anterior angulation. Fracture line (green).

Wrist

Fractures of the wrist are common and are most often caused by putting the arm out to protect oneself when falling. When there is sufficient force to produce a fracture, it will occur at the weakest part of the wrist. In teenagers and young adults, the scaphoid is the most common site. This bone is vulnerable because it bridges the proximal and distal rows of carpal bones so that stresses across it become intensified.

If a scaphoid fracture is suspected clinically, it is important to obtain a series of specific scaphoid views. This includes two oblique X-rays along with the standard AP and lateral wrist images (Figure 2.30a and b). A displaced scaphoid fracture will usually be visible on the initial X-rays, but an undisplaced fracture may not be visible, even on films repeated 2 weeks later. In this situation, MRI can be used to establish definitively whether a fracture is present (Figure 2.31a and b).

The high sensitivity of MRI for detecting fractures stems from the fact that it shows abnormalities in the medullary cavity including fracture lines and surrounding haemorrhage and oedema in the bone marrow. MRI can also reliably exclude a suspected scaphoid fracture and show if an alternative bony injury is causing the symptoms and signs.

Fractures of the distal radius can occur in any age group but are most common in the elderly due to the high prevalence of osteoporosis (Figure 2.32a and b). These injuries are often all referred to as 'Colles' fractures but the fracture which Abraham Colles specifically described is of the 'distal one-and-a-half inches of the radius with dorsal angulation and dorsal displacement'. Strictly speaking, his name should only be used for this injury and, as a general rule, for clarity it is better to describe the injury rather than name it. This enables clear communication for any given injury.

(a)

(b)

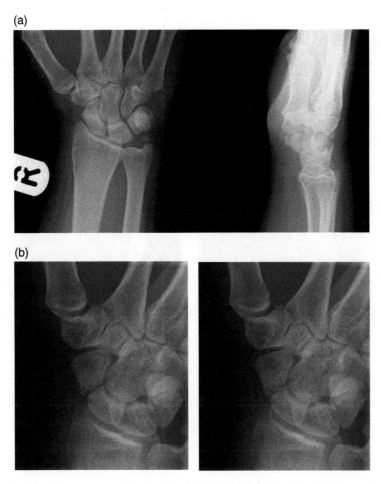

Figure 2.30 (a and b) Wrist injury in a young adult. Standard AP and lateral wrist films (a) do not show any definite bony injury but one of the additional specific scaphoid oblique views (b) demonstrate a transverse fracture across the waist of the scaphoid (orange).

(a)

(b)

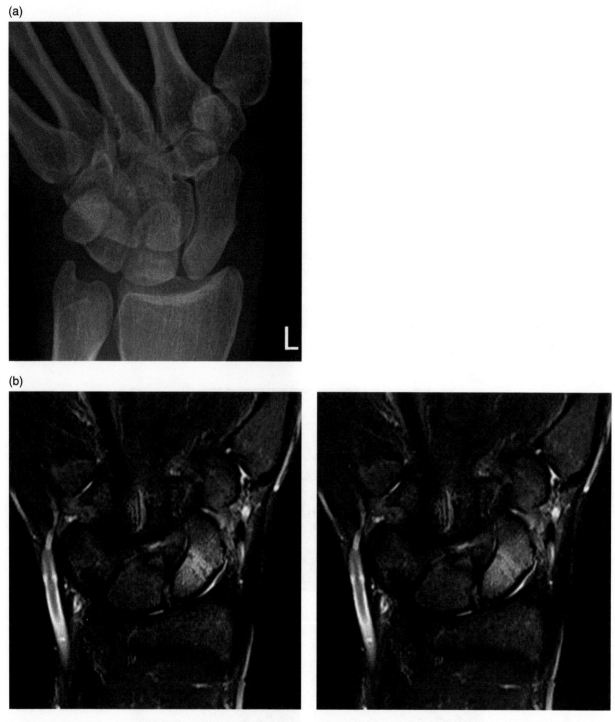

Figure 2.31 (a and b) Occult scaphoid fracture. (a) Representative image from a scaphoid series in a young adult with clinical features of a scaphoid injury. This, and the other views, shows no fracture. (b) Corresponding MRI image of the wrist demonstrating a linear fracture (blue) across the waist of the scaphoid with surrounding abnormal signal (orange) due to oedema and haemorrhage in the bone marrow.

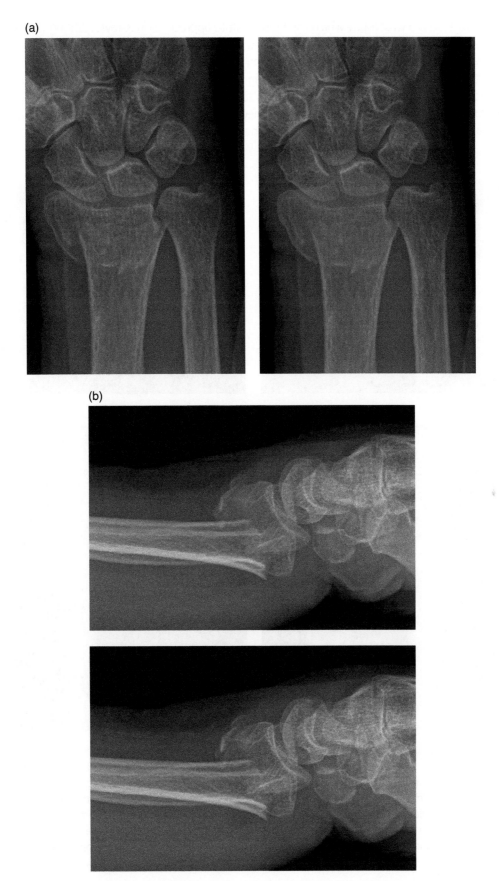

Figure 2.32 (a and b) Fracture of the distal radius in an elderly female patient. The AP view shows a transverse fracture with shortening along with lateral displacement of the distal fragment. The lateral view also shows dorsal angulation.

Perilunate dislocation is a wrist injury which can be difficult to appreciate on X-rays. Although severe disruption of the normal anatomy occurs, it can be easily overlooked unless the alignment of the carpal bones is specifically checked. One way to do this is by looking at the '4 Cs' on the lateral film (see Figure 1.5). Notice that the proximal surface of the capitate has a C shape. This sits in the C shape of the distal surface of the lunate. The proximal surface of the lunate is also C-shaped, and this sits in the fourth C, which is the distal surface of the radius. Also, compared with the normal dorsal–palmar view of the wrist, it can be seen that the lunate partially overlaps the capitate and has a more triangular appearance (Figure 2.33a and b).

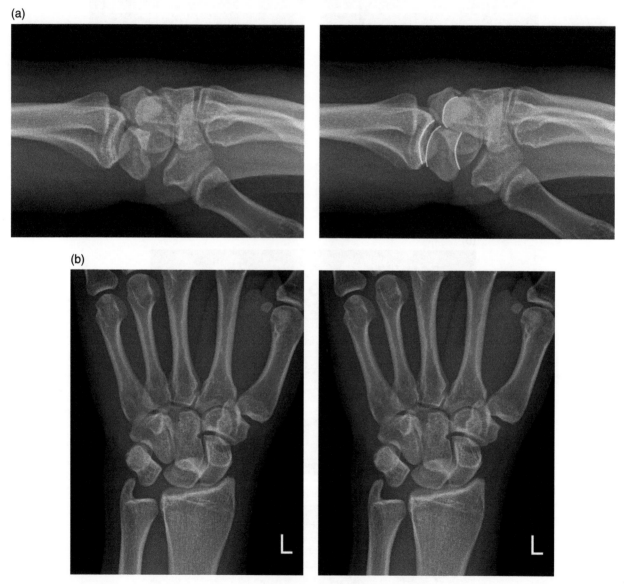

(a)

(b)

Figure 2.33 (a, lateral and b, AP): Perilunate dislocation. Signs: Although it is not easy to see because of the overlapping shadows of several different bones, the lateral view demonstrates that the distal surface of the lunate (orange) is not articulating with the proximal surface of the capitate (yellow). The latter is displaced dorsally, along with the other carpal bones, leaving just the lunate normally aligned with the radius. This is best appreciated by looking for the 'four Cs'. This row of four C-shaped articular surfaces (white) is always present on a normal lateral film. They are, moving from proximal to distal, the articular surfaces of the radius, proximal lunate, distal lunate and the capitate. On the AP film (b), the relationship of the carpal bones is also abnormal. The normally equal joint spaces around the bones are less regular, and there is an abnormal amount of overlap of the lunate with the capitate. Compare these views with the normal AP and lateral wrist in Figure 1.4.

Hip

Fractures of the femoral neck are common, particularly in the ageing population because the majority are associated with osteoporosis. It is useful to broadly separate femoral neck fractures into two groups: intra-articular and extra-articular (intertrochanteric).

An intra-articular fracture carries the risk of damaging the vessels which supply the femoral head as these run along the neck inside the joint (Figure 2.34). If there is displacement at the fracture site the vessels are likely to be torn, with a high chance of subsequent avascular necrosis (AVN) of the femoral head. Intertrochanteric fractures cross the femoral neck more distally, that is distal to the joint capsule and distal to the vessels supplying the femoral head. Therefore, there is no risk of AVN.

Treatment is aimed at allowing the patient to become pain free and mobile as quickly as possible in order to avoid complications such as bed sores, pulmonary embolus and pneumonia. Metalwork is used to replace or fix the injured part of the skeleton. Strong fixation reduces pain from the fracture site and allows the patient to begin mobilising soon after surgery.

Treatment must also take into consideration the risk of AVN. If an intra-articular fracture is minimally displaced, the vessels supplying the femoral head are likely to be intact. The femoral head is retained and the fracture fixed with canulated screws. But if the fracture is significantly displaced, the vessels supplying the femoral head are very likely to be torn and so the head is removed and replaced (Figure 2.35a and b), thus bypassing the problem of AVN. An extra-articular (intertrochanteric) fracture is fixed using a dynamic hip screw which allows compression of the fracture site while providing support across the bony injury (Figure 2.36a and b).

Displaced femoral neck fractures are usually relatively conspicuous on X-rays, but when there is no displacement they may be difficult or sometimes impossible to see. In the situation where there is clinical suspicion of a fracture but the plain films are normal, as with suspected scaphoid fractures, MRI is the investigation of choice. MRI will reliably demonstrate a femoral neck fracture if one is present, and if not, it will usually show an alternative cause for symptoms such as a pelvic insufficiency fracture or soft tissue injury (Figure 2.37a and b).

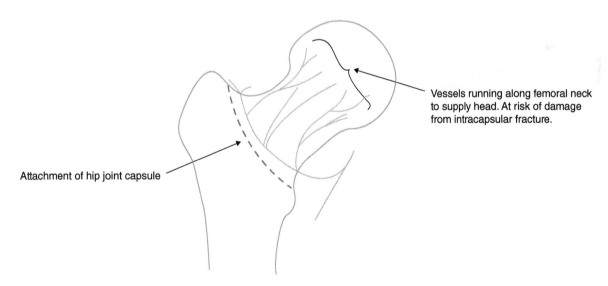

Vessels running along femoral neck to supply head. At risk of damage from intracapsular fracture.

Attachment of hip joint capsule

Figure 2.34 Diagram of blood supply to the femoral head.

(a)

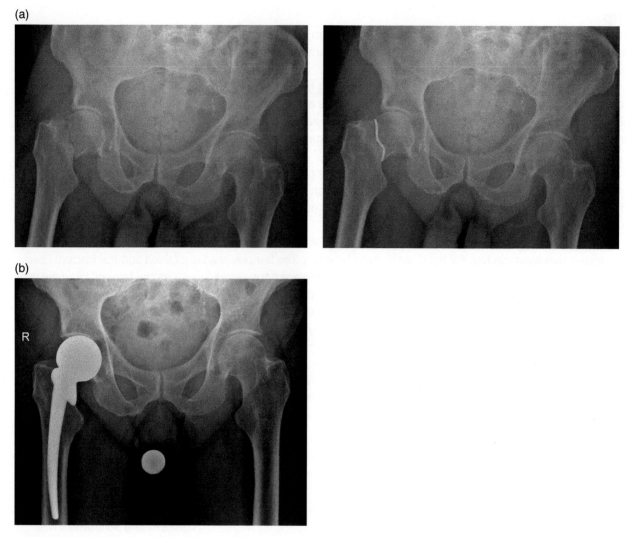

(b)

Figure 2.35 (a and b) Displaced intra-articular fracture of the right femoral neck. Signs: Fracture line across the femoral neck (yellow). Displacement: The femur has migrated proximally due to angulation at the fracture site. (b) The vessels supplying the femoral head are likely to be torn and, therefore, the best treatment is to replace the non-viable femoral head with a prosthesis, in this case a hemiarthroplasty. *Note*: The round metallic density below the pelvis in the midline on Figures 2.35b and 2.36b is a marker used to calibrate measurements of hip replacements and other implants.

(a)

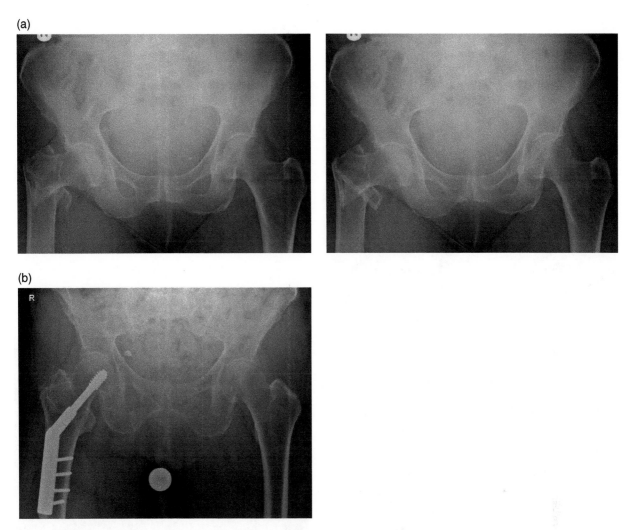

(b)

Figure 2.36 (a and b) Intertrochanteric fracture of the right femoral neck. The fracture line (orange) is distal to the joint capsule attachment and the intra-articular part of the femoral neck and therefore the vessels to the head are not at risk. (b) This fracture is treated using a dynamic hip screw to provide secure fixation and allow early mobilisation. The femoral head is retained as there is no risk of AVN.

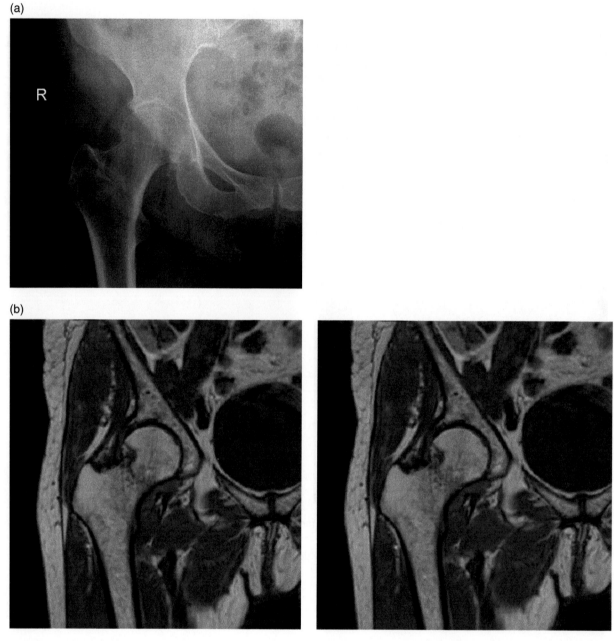

Figure 2.37 (a and b) Occult femoral neck fracture. This is a patient who has suffered a fall and has significant hip pain and cannot weight-bear. The AP film (a) shows normal appearances, as did the lateral view (not shown). MRI (b) shows a linear fracture (orange) across the bone marrow of the femoral neck.

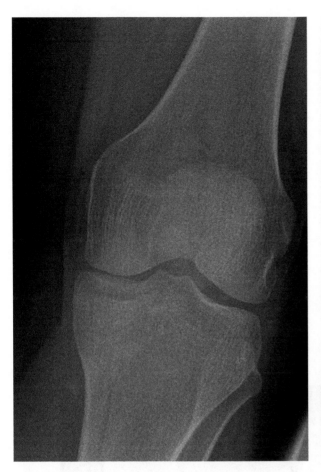
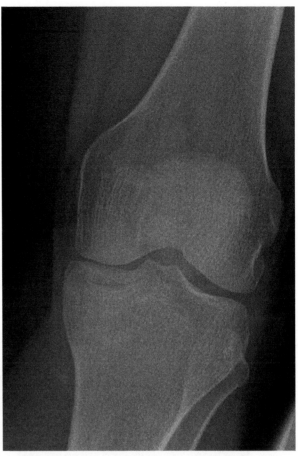

Figure 2.38 Undisplaced medial tibial plateau fracture, AP view. (The corresponding lateral film is Figure 2.23.) Signs: Linear radiolucent fracture lines are present, running horizontally in the medial tibial plateau and vertically in the proximal tibial shaft (orange).

Knee

The majority of significant knee injuries involve the soft tissue structures, the menisci and the cruciate and collateral ligaments. In this situation, X-rays often show swelling of the suprapatellar pouch but no specific signs. Clinical assessment and MRI, which directly visualises the soft tissue structures, are needed to make a specific diagnosis.

Fractures of the tibial plateau are common. They are typically seen after low-energy trauma in patients with osteoporosis (Figure 2.38) and high-energy impacts, such as traffic collisions, in those with normal bone strength. CT scanning is often used to delineate the fracture pattern fully. CT shows bone detail with high resolution, and the images can be reconstructed in multiple planes, which allows the precise location, size and orientation of fragments to be determined (Figure 2.39a and b).

Ankle and foot

There is a wide spectrum of ankle injuries varying from minor to severe (Figure 2.40a and b). It would not be possible to describe all of these here but is important to consider not only the fractures which X-rays will show but also whether there are significant soft tissue injuries accompanying these. For example, in Figure 2.40, a path of bone and soft tissue injury can be determined extending down from the fibular fracture, tearing through the interosseous membrane and then the distal tibiofibular joint (syndesmosis) before exiting via the medial malleolus fracture.

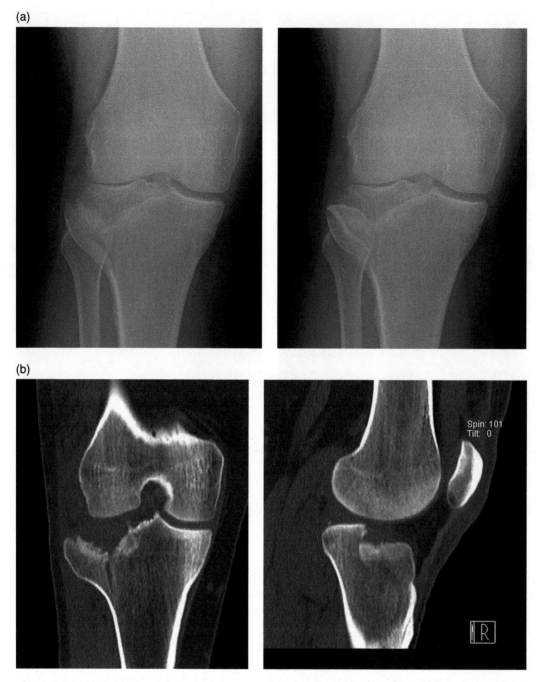

Figure 2.39 (a and b) Lateral tibial plateau fracture (blue) with severe disruption of the articular surface. AP film (a) and CT coronal and sagittal reconstructions (b). CT allows clear and accurate delineation of the bony injury. Although part of the joint surface is intact, the anterior two-thirds are severely displaced inferiorly.

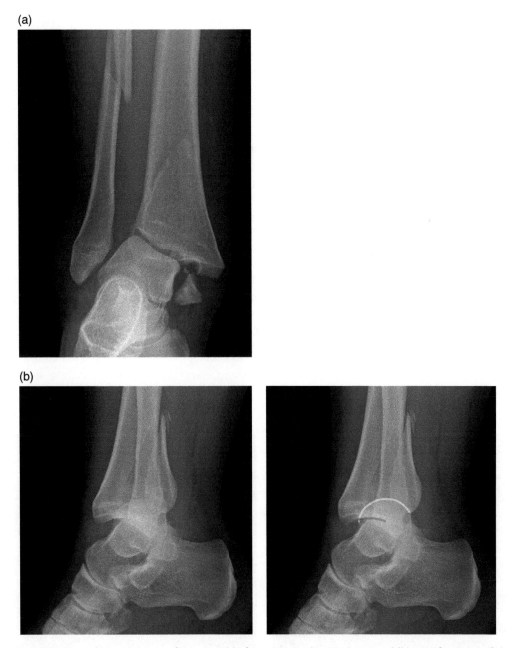

Figure 2.40 (a and b) AP and lateral X-rays of severe ankle fracture. On the AP view, in addition to fractures of the fibular shaft and medial malleolus, the space between the distal tibia and the fibula is widened, indicating disruption of the distal tibiofibular joint. The lateral view reveals a displaced fragment of bone from the posterior aspect of the distal tibia, known as the third malleolus (green), and also posterior subluxation of the talus (articular surface of tibia in orange and talus in white).

A spiral high fibular fracture is often associated with disruption of the ankle joint. The injury extends distally from the fibular fracture into the soft tissues as a tear of the interosseous membrane and then the syndesmosis between the distal tibia and fibula. The force then exits through the medial side of the ankle in the form of a tear of the ligaments or a fracture of the medial malleolus. This is also known as a *Maisonneuve fracture*. The very proximal fibular fracture may distract the patient and doctor from the ankle. Therefore, it is important to make a careful assessment of the ankle when a high fibula fracture is found.

The Lisfranc injury is a fracture–subluxation of the midfoot which is easily and commonly overlooked. It is usually caused by crushing or forced abduction of the forefoot. The bases of the lateral four metatarsals are tightly held together by strong ligaments, but these are lacking between the great and index toe metatarsal bases. As a result, trauma can produce subluxation of the lateral four tarsometatarsal joints (TMTJs). This is a severe injury in terms of soft tissue damage and can lead to chronic pain, but it is not easily seen on X-rays and consequently can be missed in emergency departments (Figure 2.41a).

Jacques **Lisfranc** de St Martin was a field surgeon in Napoleon Bonaparte's army. He did not actually describe this injury, but his name became linked with the TMTJ when, in 1815, he described 'A New Method for Performing a Partial Amputation of the Foot' through this joint as an alternative to the established treatment at the time of a more radical below-knee amputation. He was inspired to conduct his research by cases of frostbite and other injuries that he had observed on the battlefield.

The most important thing to look for on the X-ray is a change in alignment between the metatarsals and their corresponding tarsal bones. In particular, it is essential to follow the line of the medial cortex of the index metatarsal and the medial cortex of the intermediate cuneiform with which it articulates. Any step between the bones on this side of the joint is abnormal. Compare this with the normal alignment between the tarsal and the metatarsal bones (Figure 2.41b and c). There is often further evidence of injury to the TMTJs in the form of small avulsion fractures and subtle loss of the normal parallel alignment on the two sides of each TMTJ.

(a)

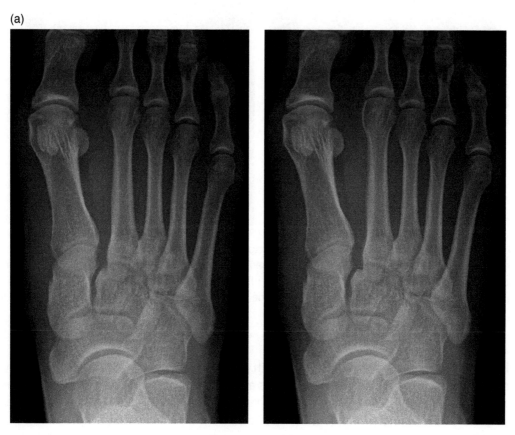

Figure 2.41

(b)

(c)

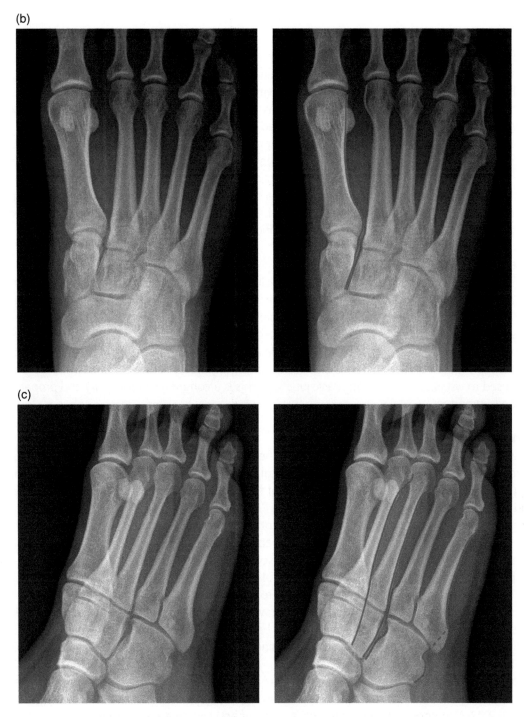

Figure 2.41 (*Continued*) (a) Lisfranc injury. The index (second) tarsometatarsal joint (TMTJ) is subluxed laterally by only 2 or 3 mm. This is shown by the step (orange) on the medial side of the index TMTJ. Although the *residual* displacement is minimal, it would have been severe as the injury occurred. Afterwards the bones have returned to a relatively normal position, disguising the fact that there is significant damage to the surrounding soft tissues. (b and c) Standard views of normal foot for comparison. By using both views, it can be seen that each metatarsal base aligns exactly with its respective tarsal bone. The exception is the styloid process of the little toe metatarsal because this is not part of the articular surface. In particular, a step where the medial border of the index metatarsal lines up with the intermediate cuneiform is abnormal.

Spine

Assessing spine X-rays

Leaving aside vertebral body insufficiency fractures, spinal injuries are most commonly seen following high-energy falls and traffic accidents. This section begins with evaluation of cervical spine X-rays, but the same principles also apply to the thoracic and lumbar regions. Patients will frequently have underlying degenerative changes in the spine and so some of the examples used include these.

Imagine taking the dry bones of a cervical spine and placing them one on top of another from C1 to C7. It would only take a small tap with the finger to send them all toppling. Therefore, the structural soft tissue components are clearly essential for maintaining resilience and integrity of the spine. These cannot be directly shown on X-rays, but it is important to think of and mentally picture these when evaluating spinal films.

The **lateral view** demonstrates the majority of cervical injuries, and therefore it is customary to look at this first. It is useful to have a mental checklist of specific features to evaluate.

Adequacy of the image

The films should show the skull base at the top and include T1 at the bottom, showing the posterior elements as well as the vertebral bodies. It is often difficult to demonstrate the cervicothoracic junction on the lateral X-ray because the bone and soft tissue of the patient's shoulders project over this area. Ways of getting round this problem include pulling on the patient's arms when the X-ray is taken or performing a 'swimmer's view' with one of the patient's arms down by their side and the other up next to their head. This depresses and elevates the shoulders, respectively, to displace the overlying tissues. If these manoeuvres are unsuccessful, CT can be used to visualise the cervicothoracic junction. This is a common site for injury and proper visualisation is important.

Alignment

Three lines can be traced on the lateral film to check the overall alignment, as shown in Figure 2.42b. For each of the three, visualise a line linking the same anatomical points on each vertebra. Each line should form a smooth curve. Look closely for any abrupt alteration of that line, in the form of either a step or a sudden change in the arc of curvature.

The anatomy of C1 and C2 differs from that of the other cervical vertebrae. C1 has lateral masses which articulate with the occipital condyles of the skull base above and the lateral masses of C2 below. In front of and behind the lateral masses of C1, the thinner bone of the anterior and posterior arches complete a bony ring. The peg extends up behind the anterior arch of C1 from the superior aspect of the body of C2 and is held against it by the transverse ligament which extends across inside the anterior part of the ring of C1. This, along with other ligamentous structures, prevents C1, along with the head, from sliding forwards and backwards and so prevents damage to the spinal cord, which lies behind the peg in the vertebral canal. If the transverse ligament is ruptured, the peg of C2 is no longer restrained and the space between the peg and the anterior arch of C1 may widen.

The relationship between the anterior arch of C1 and the odontoid peg of C2 is checked on the lateral view by measuring the space between these structures. In adults, this gap should be 2 mm or less at the narrowest point (Figure 2.42b). In normal children, the 'space' is wider and can measure up to 5 mm.

As part of assessing alignment, check that the end plates of the vertebral bodies either side of each disc space are parallel to one another and that the articular surfaces at each facet joint are parallel on the two sides of each joint. Also look to see that the spacing of the spinous processes is even with no abrupt widening (Figure 2.42c).

Bones

Check each cervical vertebra for any fracture, following the anterior and posterior elements carefully. Look at the vertebral body height and shape for any deformity, as well as searching for any fracture lines of the vertebral bodies and posterior elements.

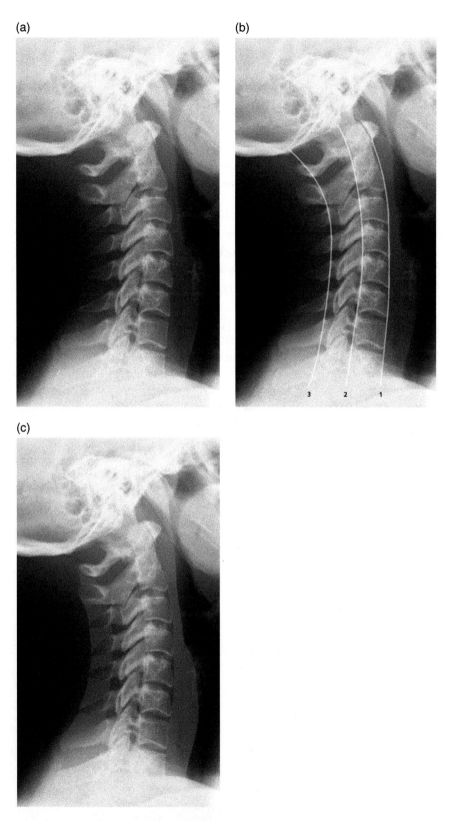

(a)

(b)

(c)

Figure 2.42 (a, b and c) Assessing the lateral c-spine film. (b) Line 1 follows the anterior cortex of the vertebral bodies, although not including C1 due to the different anatomical arrangement at this level. Line 2 follows the posterior cortex of the vertebral bodies, also extending up along the posterior aspect of the peg of C2. Line 3 is called the spinolaminar line because it runs along the bases of the spinous processes, where these join the laminae. All three lines should be smooth curves with no step or abrupt change in curvature. The space between the anterior arch of C1 and the peg of C2 (green) should measure 2 mm or less at its narrowest point in an adult. (c) Look for even spacing between the adjacent vertebrae at the discs, facet joints and spinous processes. The spaces between the latter (orange) are occupied by the interspinous ligaments. The prevertebral soft tissue shadow (green) should also be assessed.

Anterior soft tissues

Some, but not all, cervical spine injuries are accompanied by enough anterior soft tissue swelling to cause visible widening on the lateral film. The prevertebral soft tissue thickness can be assessed on a lateral X-ray because their anterior aspect is demarcated by air in the pharynx, down to C4, and air in the trachea below this level. As a general rule for adults, the soft tissue thickness should not exceed 7 mm at the C2 level and 22 mm at the C6 level. Measurements vary in children and also change with swallowing and other factors and should be considered as a clue rather than definitive evidence of significant injury (Figure 2.42c).

AP views

Take a similar approach to the lateral view. Assess alignment by checking that the spinous processes, which are often bifid, form a straight vertical line with no sudden change in direction or in their spacing (Figure 2.43). Also make sure the lateral cortex of each vertebral body lines up with those above and below. Do the same for the pedicles and facet joints. Check the bones for fracture lines and for deformity such as reduced height of a vertebral body.

The alignment between C1 and C2 also needs to be checked from the frontal direction. This area is hidden by the overlying mandible and other structures on the straight AP view, so a specific view is performed through the open mouth (Figure 2.44). On this view, check if the outer margins of the lateral masses of C1 above and those of C2 below are aligned with one another (a step of up to 2 mm can be within normal limits here). Also the space between the peg of C2 and the lateral masses of C1 should be equal on both sides. Head rotation can cause asymmetry, so make sure the patient's head is not rotated, by checking that the gap between the incisor teeth is in the midline on this film. A common C1 injury is the burst fracture where force on the top of the head forces the lateral masses of C1 apart, causing the anterior and posterior arches to fracture. This shows on the through-mouth view as lateral displacement of the C1 lateral masses so that they no longer align

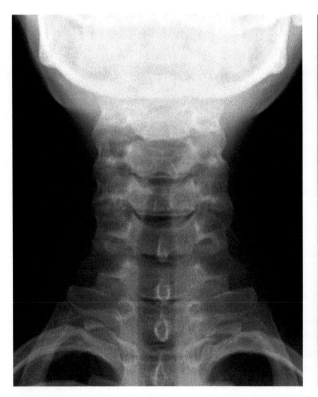 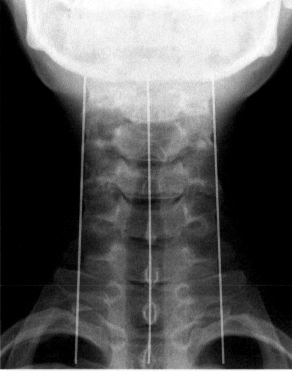

Figure 2.43 Normal cervical spine, AP view: Straight alignment and spacing of the spinous processes (orange) should be checked. There should be no abrupt alteration of either. Also the lateral borders of the vertebrae should align with one another.

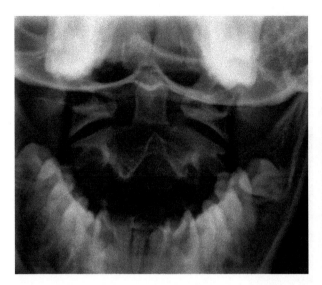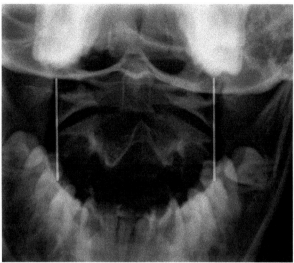

Figure 2.44 Normal through-mouth view of C1 and C2. In addition to looking for fracture lines, check symmetrical spacing of the peg of C2 with the lateral masses of C1 (green). Also the lateral sides of the lateral masses of C1 must align with those of C2 (white lines). A step of 2 mm or more is abnormal.

with those of C2. Next, inspect the bones themselves carefully for fracture lines or deformity, particularly looking for fractures of the odontoid peg.

Figures 2.45, 2.46, 2.47a and b and 2.48 show examples of cervical spine injuries.

Increasingly, CT scanning is now used as a first-line investigation for suspected spinal trauma. It provides extremely good bone detail, and images can be reconstructed in any plane. As a result, subtle fractures can be detected and their precise configuration shown (Figure 2.48c). In addition, it can be combined with scanning other areas of the body such as the head, chest, abdomen and pelvis for patients with multiple injuries.

MRI has an important role in imaging the spine of patients with a neurological deficit following injury as it is able to directly demonstrate the cord and spinal nerve roots (Figure 2.47c).

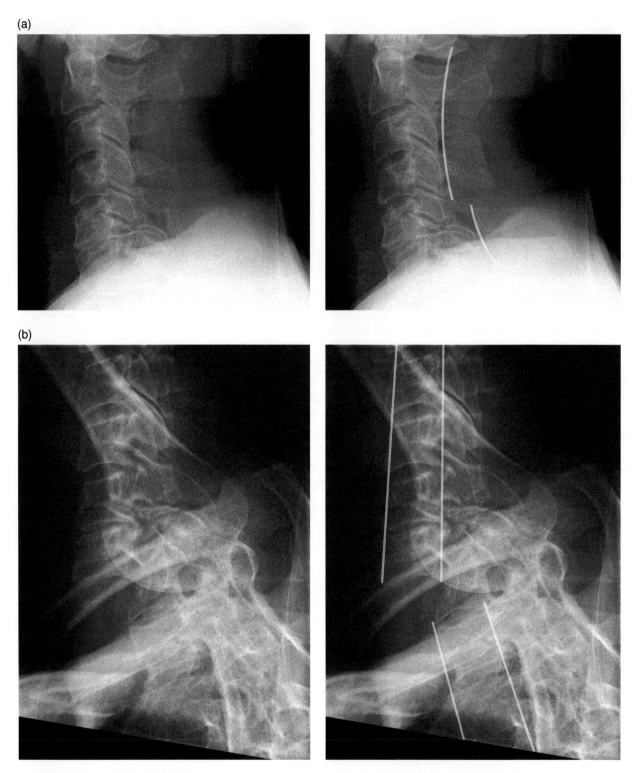

Figure 2.45 (a and b) A patient with severe lower c-spine subluxation from a high-force traffic injury. Assessing the adequacy of the first film reveals that it demonstrates the vertebrae down to C6 only. A second lateral image performed as a 'swimmer's view' shows the cervicothoracic junction more fully. Alignment at C6/7 is grossly abnormal. A combination of the two views shows that all three of the lines discussed in Figure 2.42b are abnormal and that the bodies of C6 and C7 are separated. Also the regular spacing between the spinous processes (orange) changes at the injured level (red).

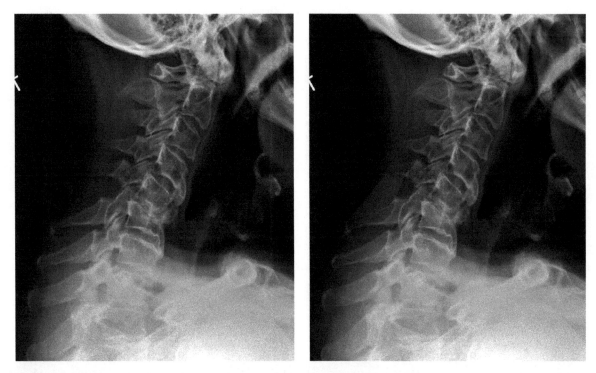

Figure 2.46 Fracture of the body of C6 with anterior wedging plus separation of the spinous processes of C5 and C6, indicating rupture of the interspinous and supraspinus ligaments, which usually hold these together. Vertebral body fracture (green). Enlarged space between spinous processes (orange). Although this patient has prominent osteophytes, these should be ignored when following the line along the anterior aspect of the vertebral bodies. Following the lines shown in Figure 2.42b shows an abrupt change in angulation of the three lines.

(a)

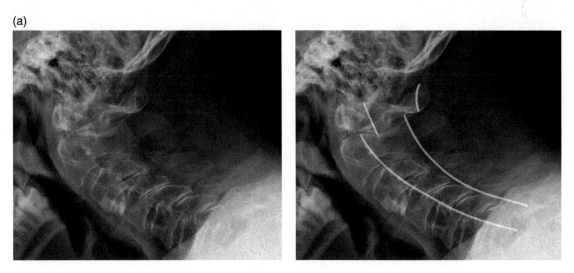

Figure 2.47 (a and b) Fracture of the base of the peg of C2. The posterior cortex of the peg is displaced backwards relative to the posterior cortex of its vertebral body. C1 has displaced backwards along with the peg, and therefore the spinolaminar line shows abrupt posterior displacement at this level.

(b)

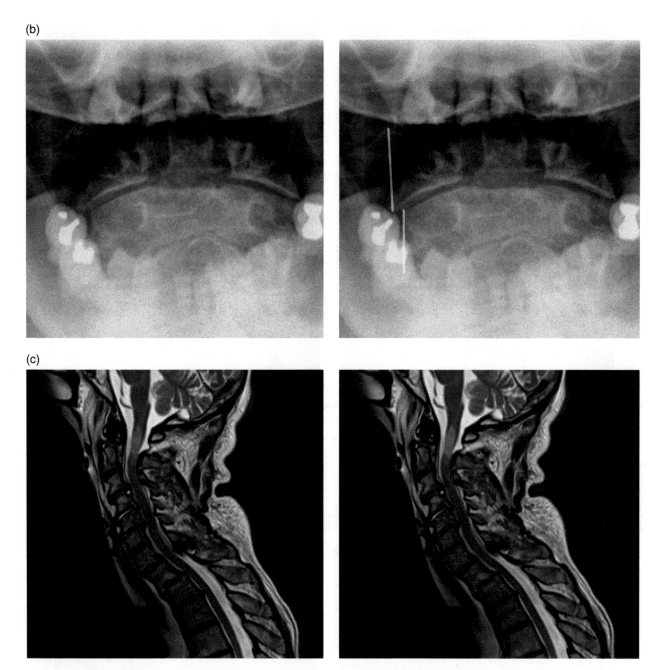

(c)

Figure 2.47 (b) The through-mouth view shows the fracture (orange on both views). In addition, there is a further injury of C1. Its lateral masses are displaced outwards relative to those of C2. This means that the ring of C1 is abnormally wide, and therefore a 'burst' fracture is present. (c) MRI of the patient (as shown in Figure 2.47a and b) scanned due to clinical features of cord injury: There is altered signal indicating contusion in the substance of the cord at the level of the C1/2 injury (orange).

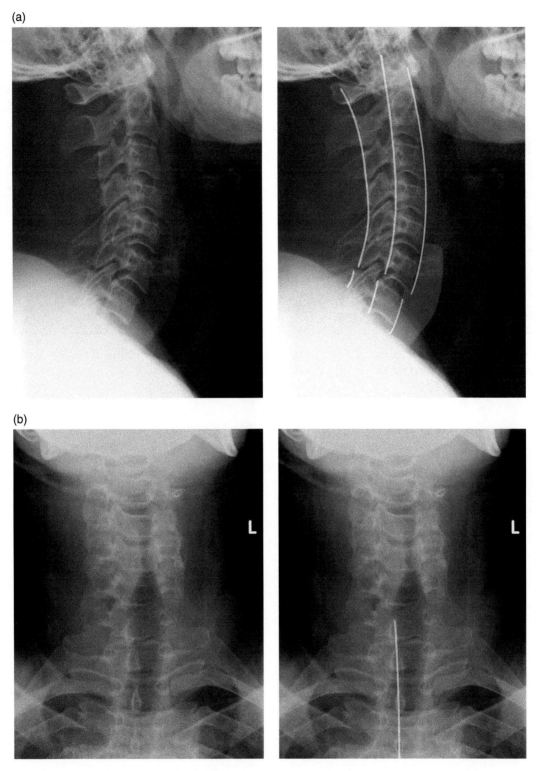

Figure 2.48 (a, b and c) Unilateral fracture/subluxation of C6/7. The lateral X-ray (a) shows subtle alteration of alignment and prevertebral soft tissue swelling (green) at the level of injury. The AP film (b) shows a change in alignment of the spinous processes (orange). Above C7, these are displaced to the right rather than continuing in the midline. They are not clearly visible because they are projected over the other lateral bony structures. A sagittal CT reconstruction through the right-sided facet joints.

(c)

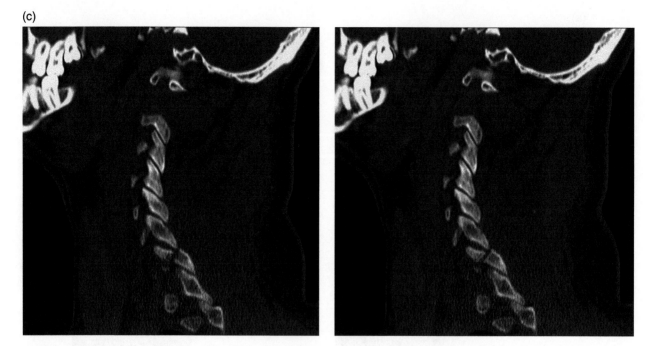

Figure 2.48 (c) Shows an occult fracture of C7 (red), extending from the superior to the inferior articular process. C6 has slipped anteriorly relative to the posterior elements below.

Paediatric fractures

The paediatric skeleton differs from the adult's, and this has a bearing on both the X-ray appearances and also some of the injuries which occur.

In children, the normal features of ongoing bone growth may add to the difficulty of X-ray interpretation. These include areas of partially or completely unossified cartilage. As cartilage has the same density as adjacent soft tissue, it cannot be directly visualised on a plain X-ray. Growth plates and synchondroses can mimic fractures. The normal growth plate undulates smoothly as it runs across the bone, and the proximal and distal surfaces are outlined by fine sclerotic margins. For example, see the distal radius growth plate (distal to the fracture) in Figure 2.52. This differs from how a fracture line crossing the bone might appear as an acute fracture lacks sclerotic margins. These features are found at various anatomical sites at specific ages, so becoming familiar with some of the more commonly confusing ones is helpful (e.g. Figures 2.49, 2.50, and 2.51).

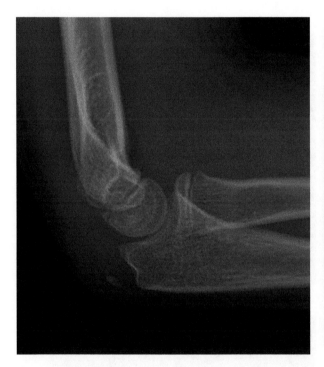 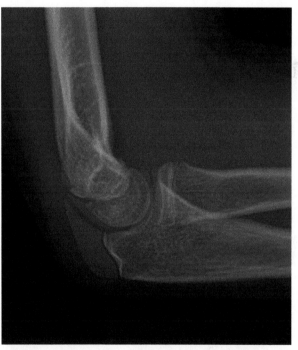

Figure 2.49 A child's elbow is identical in shape to an adult's, but a lot of the bone consists of cartilage which has not yet ossified (orange). Cartilage has the same X-ray density as the surrounding soft tissues making it essentially invisible on plain films. It can be shown using ultrasound or MRI however. Also note the appearances of the growth plates (green), with their smooth undulations and corticated outline.

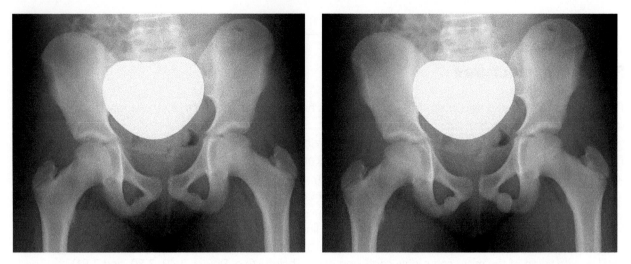

Figure 2.50 Normal synchondroses in a child (green). The temporary localised bone thickening is part of the normal growth process but can be mistaken for healing fractures.

(a)

(b)

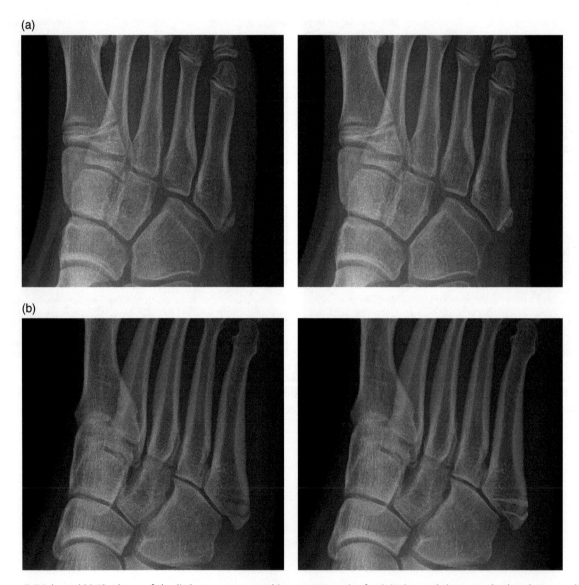

Figure 2.51 (a and b) The base of the little toe metacarpal is a common site for injuries and the growth plate here can be mistaken for a fracture. However, (a) the growth plate (yellow) always has a longitudinal orientation, whereas (b) a fracture tends to run transversely (orange). Also note the smooth rounded appearance of the margins of the growth plate compared with the sharp, uncorticated edges of the fracture.

Children's bones are less brittle than adults' with the result that fractures sometimes cause a buckle in the cortex rather than a clean break (Figure 2.52).

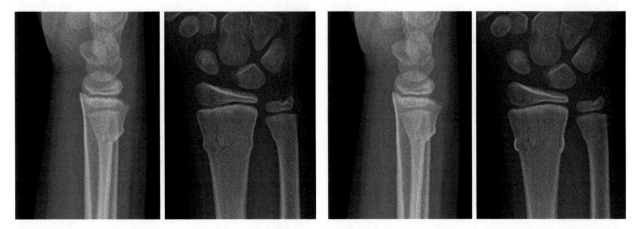

Figure 2.52 A buckle or torus fracture of the distal radial metaphysis in a child. Signs: The dorsal, medial and lateral sides of the bone have buckled slightly at the fracture site, deforming the normally smooth curve of the cortex. The lack of sharp fracture margins, which would be seen in an adult, reflects the less brittle nature of the paediatric skeleton.

In addition, growth plates are sites of relative weakness so that injuries in these areas have a tendency to extend partially or completely along them (Figures 2.53, 2.54 and 2.55).

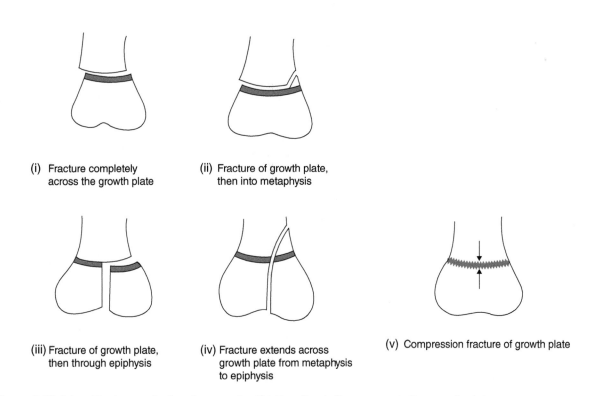

(i) Fracture completely across the growth plate

(ii) Fracture of growth plate, then into metaphysis

(iii) Fracture of growth plate, then through epiphysis

(iv) Fracture extends across growth plate from metaphysis to epiphysis

(v) Compression fracture of growth plate

Figure 2.53 Salter–Harris growth plate fracture classification. Purple line represents the growth plate.

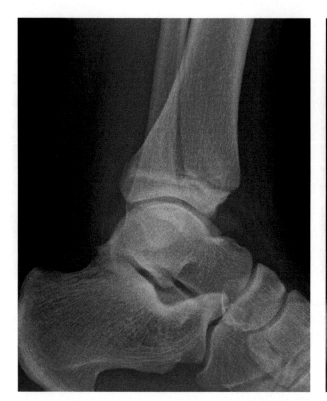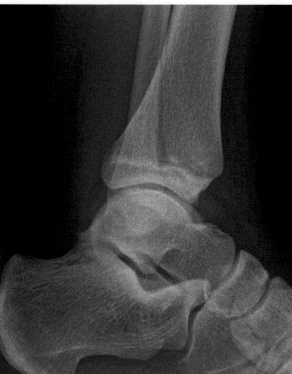

Figure 2.54 Salter–Harris II fracture of the distal tibia in an adolescent. The fracture line (orange) extends partially along the growth plate and then superiorly across a corner of the metaphysis.

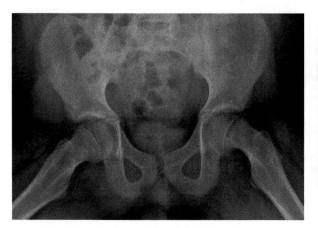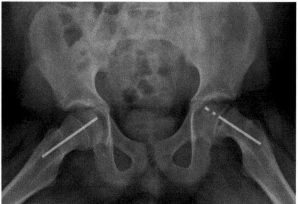

Figure 2.55 Slipped upper left femoral epiphysis: A 13-year-old boy with left hip pain following a minor hip injury. In this condition, the proximal femoral epiphysis slips *posteriorly* at the growth plate. The displacement is therefore difficult to see on an AP film and is best seen on a lateral view of the upper femur. This is achieved by asking the patient to rotate both knees outwards, which externally rotates the femurs. On the normal, right side, a line drawn up through the centre of the femoral neck extends through the centre of the femoral epiphysis, but on the left the femoral head does not lie centrally on the neck and therefore has slipped.

Slipped upper femoral epiphysis is the most common significant cause for hip pain in the age group of 10–15 years.

A 'frog lateral' X-ray (Figure 2.55) should always be obtained for children of this age range. The epiphysis slides posteriorly relative to the metaphysis making the abnormality inconspicuous on a standard AP film.

Obesity and endocrine disorders are predisposing factors.

Supracondylar fracture of the humerus

Supracondylar fractures of the humerus are a common injury in children. They are usually associated with posterior angulation of the distal fragment, and when displacement is moderate or severe, the injury is easy to spot (Figure 2.56a and b). However, a minimally displaced fracture may be difficult to diagnose. In this situation, the 'anterior humeral line sign' can be very helpful. Using the lateral film, a line is drawn down the anterior cortex of the distal humeral shaft. When this is extended towards the elbow, it should normally pass through the middle third of the capitellum. (In young children, this may only be visible as an ossification centre rather than a fully visible ossified structure.) If the distal part of the humerus, including the capitellum, is angled backwards after a fracture, the line passes anterior to the middle third of the capitellum (Figure 2.57).

(a)

(b)

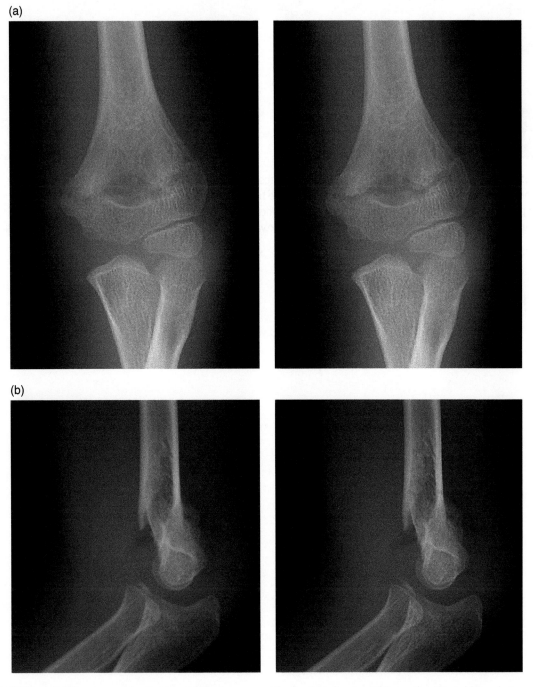

Figure 2.56 (a and b) Supracondylar fracture of the humerus. The fracture line is visible on the AP and lateral views (orange), and the lateral also shows the typical posterior angulation of the distal fragment.

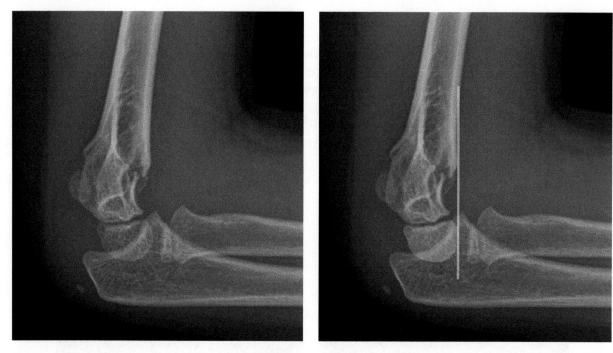

Figure 2.57 In this second patient with a less displaced supracondylar fracture, the anterior humeral line sign helps confirm the diagnosis. A line is drawn down the anterior cortex of the humeral shaft. When this is extended distally, it should normally pass through the middle third of the capitellum ossification centre (blue). However, in this patient, posterior angulation at the fracture site has shifted the capitellum backwards, causing the line to pass anterior to the capitellum.

Fractures in child abuse

The diagnosis of non-accidental injury (NAI) is complex and depends on evidence collected from all agencies involved in the care of the child. In the case of children who have been physically injured by a carer, X-rays play an important role in the detection of fractures and the assessment of specific patterns of trauma. Once it is thought that a child has been deliberately injured, care and investigation should be delivered by consultants in paediatrics and radiology. These investigations include a skeletal survey to allow the detection of occult bony injuries, obtain further information about a clinically suspected injury and aid in the dating of bone injuries. It may also help in the diagnosis of any underlying skeletal disorder which may predispose to fractures.

There are times when NAI may have not been initially suspected, for example an incidental rib fracture found on a chest X-ray performed for chest infection or when the injury shown on an X-ray is not consistent with the history given by the carer. Therefore, it is a good idea to have an understanding of some key concepts and possible X-ray findings.

The diagnosis can be missed if NAI is not considered, in which case the child is at a high risk of repeated abuse that may be fatal. Up to half of fatally abused children have been seen within the previous month by a healthcare professional. Investigations into those cases where the opportunity to intervene has been missed emphasise how important it is to clearly communicate any suspicion of NAI between relevant professionals. For a trainee doctor, this will usually mean discussion with a senior paediatrician at the earliest possible opportunity. Child protection is everyone's responsibility, but the recognition of subtle injuries requires experience in the radiological features of paediatric trauma – both accidental and non-accidental – and therefore suspected abnormalities should always be discussed with an experienced radiologist. The X-ray findings, as always, have to be considered in the overall clinical context. For example, physical abuse should be considered when an infant presents with a fracture in the absence of a history of significant trauma or a known medical condition that predisposes to bone fragility.

Risk factors

Pre-mobile children are less prone to accidental injury, so the younger the child the more likely the fracture to be inflicted.
Skeletal injuries from abuse are more common in younger children, that is infants and toddlers (<3 years). Children with disabilities are also at increased risk of abuse.

X-ray features

The pattern of fractures is important. Multiple fractures of different ages without an adequate explanation are highly suggestive of NAI, especially if present on both sides of the body.

Some types of fracture are more specific for NAI than others. For example, metaphyseal fractures, as described later, and rib fractures have high specificity. Fractures of the digits have moderate specificity. Long bone shaft fractures have lower specificity.

Metaphyseal fractures
This type of fracture extends through the metaphysis immediately adjacent to the growth plate, where the bone is relatively weak (Figure 2.58). Depending on the angle of the X-ray beam relative to the fracture line, they have a 'corner' or 'bucket handle'

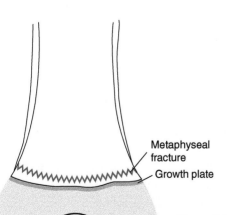

Metaphyseal fracture

Growth plate

Figure 2.58 Diagrammatic representation of metaphyseal fracture. The injury occurs immediately adjacent to the growth plate and extends transversely across the bone, separating a disc-shaped fragment. On an X-ray, this fragment may have the appearance of a 'bucket handle' or 'corner' depending on the angle of the X-ray.

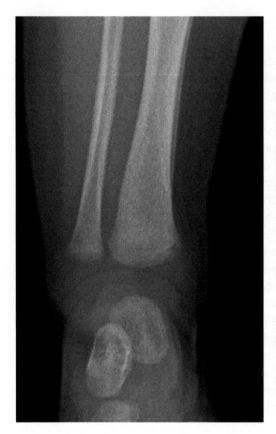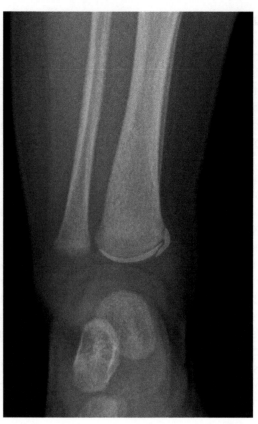

Figure 2.59 AP X-ray of the distal tibia of a 2-month-old child showing a metaphyseal fracture caused by child abuse. The fracture runs just proximal to the growth plate, with the separated fragment of metaphysis giving the impression of a 'bucket handle' (yellow). (The distal tibial epiphysis is not visible at this age as its ossification centre has not yet appeared.)

appearance (Figure 2.59). Metaphyseal fractures may result from a violent pulling or twisting of a limb or from the limb flailing violently when a child is shaken and are a characteristic feature of NAI because of the nature of the external force needed to produce such an injury. However, the clinical context remains important. For example, a difficult delivery may also cause metaphyseal (and other) fractures (Figure 2.60).

Rib fractures are usually caused by compression of the chest, often in the AP direction when a child is picked up and squeezed with a high degree of force. They are subtle and difficult to diagnose but should be carefully sought. Look for posterior fractures in the paraspinal region as well as the more anterior parts of the ribs. Like undisplaced rib fractures in any patient, they are commonly not visible until callus develops and gives the fracture site a focally expanded appearance (Figure 2.61). Oblique and delayed X-rays help to increase the sensitivity of detection.

Features associated with possible child abuse

The following indicators can be used to inform decisions about the likelihood of child abuse:
- Multiple fractures are more common after physical abuse than after non-abusive traumatic injury.
- A child with multiple rib fractures has a 7 in 10 chance of having been abused.
- A child with a femoral fracture has a 1 in 3–4 chance of having been abused.
- Femoral fractures resulting from abuse are more commonly seen in children who are not yet walking.
- A child aged under 3 years with a humeral fracture has a 1 in 2 chance of having been abused.
- Mid-shaft fractures of the humerus are more common in abuse than in non-abuse, whereas supracondylar fractures are more likely to have non-abusive causes.
- An infant or a toddler with a skull fracture has a 1 in 3 chance of having been abused.
  Source: BMJ (2008). Reproduced with permission of BMJ Publishing Ltd.

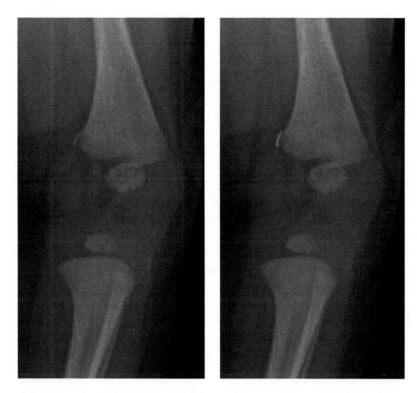

Figure 2.60 AP X-ray of the knee of an infant. There is a 'corner' fracture of the medial aspect of the distal femoral metaphysis (yellow). This type of injury is caused by traction and twisting forces, and so is frequently associated with child abuse. However, in this case, it was the result of a difficult delivery. This emphasises the importance of correlating the history and other information fully.

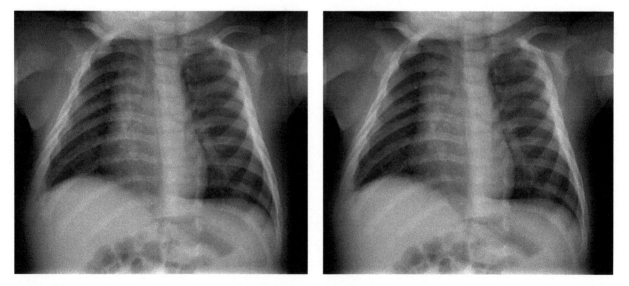

Figure 2.61 Chest X-ray of a 2-month-old child. There are healing fractures of the right 4th and 11th ribs posteriorly, caused by child abuse. These are visible because callus produces subtle focal thickening of the ribs at the fracture sites (orange).

Other imaging modalities

X-rays are an accurate first-line investigation in skeletal injury. To get the most from them, it is necessary to be aware of the significance of both bony and soft tissue signs, which may be subtle. It is also important to be aware of the limitations of plain X-rays and to make use of alternative imaging tests when they can provide additional help.

When fractures are complicated, CT is often useful to show the position and size of the fragments. The limb is scanned in the transverse plane, and the data can then be processed to produce images in the coronal, sagittal or any other plane. CT can also create a 3D image of the bony anatomy.

MRI is widely used for evaluating injuries of the soft tissues, including intra-articular damage in the knee and other joints. It is also very accurate for detecting or excluding occult bony injuries, such as undisplaced femoral neck or scaphoid fractures and insufficiency fractures of the sacrum and pubic rami. In the spine, it can again reveal occult fractures and can directly visualise individual nerve roots and the spinal cord itself, as well as structural soft tissue elements.

Ultrasound also allows high-resolution imaging of certain soft tissue injuries. It is particularly useful for evaluating tendons, in areas such as the shoulder, the wrist and the Achilles tendon.

Further reading

1. Kemp, Alison M; Dunstan, Frank; Harrison, Sara; Morris, Susan; Mann, Mala; Rolfe, Kim; Datta, Shalini; Thomas, D Phillip; Sibert, Jonathan R; Maguire, Sabine 2008. Patterns of skeletal fractures in child abuse: systematic review. BMJ; 337: a1518.
2. Royal College of Radiologists/Royal College of Paediatrics and Child Health. *Standards for radiological investigations of suspected non-accidental injury*. London: Royal College of Paediatrics and Child Health, 2008. Available at: www.rcr.ac. uk/docs/radiology/pdf/RCPCH_RCR_final.pdf (accessed on 19 September 2014).

3 Arthritis

Osteoarthritis

Osteoarthritis (OA) is the most common form of arthropathy. Articular cartilage becomes damaged and thinned, followed by changes in the adjacent bone. Bony proliferation occurs, producing osteophytes plus sclerosis and cysts in the subchondral bone. There are many factors involved in the pathophysiology, particularly genetic and environmental influences, and inflammation triggered in the joint capsule by products from the damaged cartilage is thought to have a key role. Some authors prefer the term osteoarthrosis as they think that these inflammatory changes (i.e. 'arthritis') are not necessarily a primary feature of the condition but recent research proposes a more significant role for inflammation in the pathophysiology of this condition.

OA is often described as a 'wear, tear and repair' process, and any cause of stressful loading across a joint, such as a previous injury to the articular surface or obesity, can be precipitating factors. As well as these local influences, systemic abnormalities of articular cartilage can predispose to OA. For example, it is seen more frequently in diabetes and acromegaly.

Typical patient
An elderly person complaining of gradually worsening toothache-type pain and stiffness in the hip or knee with reduced range of movement and walking distance due to pain.

Distribution

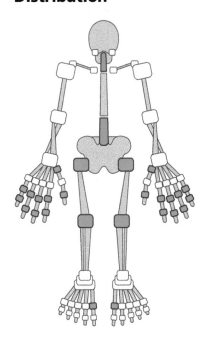

OA may be an monoarthritis (single joint affected), oligoarthritis (less than five joints) or polyarthritis (many joints), typically involving the finger distal interphalangeal (DIP), proximal interphalangeal (PIP), thumb carpometacarpal (CMC), great toe metatarsophalangeal (MTP) joints, axial skeleton, and large weight bearing joint of the hips and knees.

Musculoskeletal X-rays for Medical Students and Trainees, First Edition. Andrew K. Brown and David G. King.
© 2017 John Wiley & Sons, Ltd. Published 2017 by John Wiley & Sons, Ltd.

Clinical practice points

An X-ray is the standard first-line investigation in the assessment of OA.

X-ray signs of OA may all be present together in the same joint but often only some features will be visible.

Areas of articular cartilage damage may be severe but focal rather than affecting a whole joint surface. In this situation, the overall joint space may be preserved and therefore appear normal on X-rays, despite significant damage.

At the knee, weight-bearing films taken with the patient standing will give a more accurate picture of cartilage loss and joint deformity. For example, a patient with severe medial compartment OA may have normal joint alignment when supine, changing to a valgus knee with loss of medial joint space when the patient stands.

It is estimated that OA causes joint pain in 8.5 million people in the UK (NHS evidence).

OA is the main indication for joint replacement surgery.

Risk factors for OA include advancing age, female sex, positive family history, obesity, oestrogen deficiency, previous trauma, pre-existing joint abnormality and occupation.

There can be a wide variation in severity and natural history, and often X-ray appearances will not necessarily correlate with a patient's symptoms.

A number of scoring systems have been developed in an attempt to objectively classify the severity of OA, for example *Kellgren and Lawrence*:

- **Grade 0:** Normal
- **Grade 1:** Doubtful, that is possible narrowing of the joint space and osteophytes
- **Grade 2:** Minimal, that is mild narrowing of the joint space and small osteophytes
- **Grade 3:** Moderate, that is definite joint space narrowing, multiple moderately sized osteophytes, some subchondral sclerotic areas and possible deformity of the bone contour
- **Grade 4:** Severe, that is marked joint space narrowing, multiple large osteophytes, marked subchondral sclerosis and definite deformity of the bone contour

---

X-ray features

- **Joint space narrowing** – this reflects reduction in thickness of the articular cartilage. This may be localised and asymmetrical (unlike inflammatory arthritis, e.g. rheumatoid arthritis (RA)).
- **Osteophytes** – these are seen as small bony outgrowths at the margins of the articular surfaces of the affected joint. They can be particularly prominent at the great toe metatarsophalangeal joint (MTPJ), leading to the condition of hallux rigidus, in which the range of movement at the great toe becomes severely restricted.
- **Subchondral sclerosis** – increased density of the bone immediately below the articular cartilage.
- **Subchondral cysts** – rounded lucent areas in the subchondral bone.
- **Secondary signs** – additional features seen on X-rays in OA include signs of joint swelling (see section 'Introduction'), abnormal alignment such as varus or valgus deformity and ossified bodies in or adjacent to the joint (particularly with elbow OA). As the condition progresses, there may be bone remodelling, deformity or ankylosis.

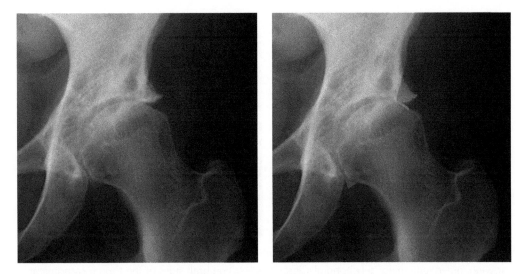

Figure 3.1 Features of OA with marginal osteophytes (purple) and supero-lateral joint space narrowing (green). The adjacent subchondral bone of the acetabulum shows areas of increased density (sclerosis) relative to normal bone and rounded areas of reduced density due to the presence of a subchondral cyst (blue).

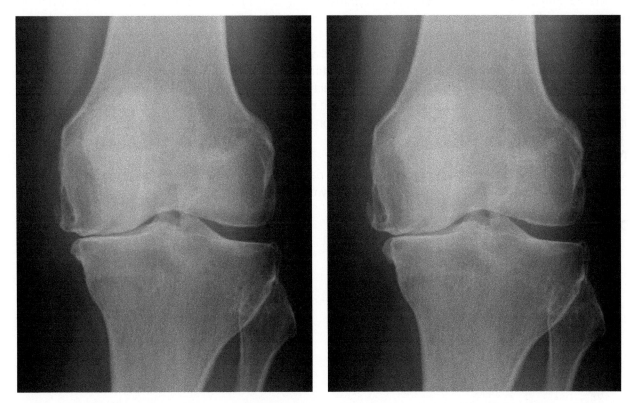

Figure 3.2 Osteoarthritis (OA) of the knee. Moderately severe OA changes are present in the medial compartment in the form of joint space narrowing (green) and marginal osteophytes (purple).

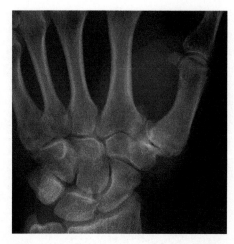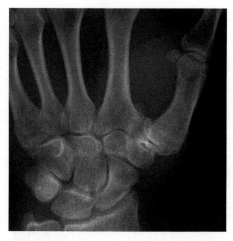

Figure 3.3 Osteoarthritis (OA) of the first carpometacarpal joint. Typical OA changes with prominent osteophytes (purple), joint space narrowing (green) and minor subchondral sclerosis (yellow) on both sides of the thumb carpometacarpal joint.

Rheumatoid arthritis

RA is the most common type of inflammatory polyarthritis. It is a chronic systemic autoimmune disease causing synovial inflammation and is characterised by a symmetrical deforming peripheral joint polyarthritis which may be associated with the development of subcutaneous nodules and multi-system manifestations.

It is important to identify RA early and refer promptly for specialist assessment by a Rheumatologist. This is because early diagnosis and rapid and aggressive suppression and tight control of inflammation improves patient outcomes by relieving symptoms of joint pain, stiffness and swelling; reducing the likelihood of permanent joint damage; maintaining function and quality of life and preventing permanent disability. Fortunately in the majority of patients, this inflammation is treatable with modern drug therapies and targeted approaches to treatment, meaning that disease remission in RA is now an achievable target.

Typical patient
A middle-aged patient complaining of gradual onset of pain and morning stiffness and swelling affecting joints in the fingers, wrists and toes (and maybe others) in a symmetrical distribution.

Distribution

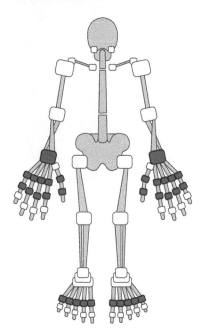

RA is typically a polyarthritis affecting the small joints of the hands (MCP and PIPs), feet (MTPs and PIPs) and wrists in a symmetrical distribution.

Clinical practice points

X-rays remain the standard method of assessing joint damage in RA, even though they are not as sensitive as cross-sectional imaging such as ultrasound or MRI at detecting signs of inflammatory arthritis. Indeed, X-rays may be normal in up to 70% of patients presenting to an early arthritis clinic despite clinical features suggestive of an early inflammatory arthritis, and characteristic radiographic signs are often only visible in patients with more established disease.

Although all patients with RA should receive a baseline X-ray of the joints of their hands, wrists and feet, radiographic abnormalities are not essential to make the diagnosis of RA and indeed modern management aims to prevent these from developing.

Assessment of radiographic joint damage remains an important outcome measure in RA to assess disease progression and response to treatment. There are many validated scoring systems to objectively quantify erosions and joint space narrowing, for example Sharp and Larson scores, which are mostly used in clinical trials. In routine clinical practice, typically patients have X-rays taken of the hand and feet joints every 12–24 months.

The most common sites for erosive changes in RA are the radial aspect of the second MCP joint, ulnar aspect of the fifth MCPJ, ulnar styloid at the wrist and lateral border of the fifth metatarsophalangeal (MTP) joint, so these areas on an X-ray should be studied in particular detail.

The cervical spine should always be considered as part of the radiological assessment of RA and may be affected in up to 80% of patients with established disease. Inflammation at the atlanto-axial joint can lead to joint damage and possibly subluxation with spinal cord and brainstem compression.

In the UK, 1 in 100 people have RA.

Untreated RA can result in significant morbidity, for example physical disability and job loss and reduced life expectancy, and has significant personal and societal costs.

Uncontrolled chronic systemic inflammation can not only permanently damage joints but can also result in osteoporosis, sarcopenia, insulin resistance, premature atherosclerosis and early ischaemic heart disease.

X-ray features

- **Soft tissue swelling** – increased soft tissue shadowing may be visible reflecting synovial inflammation.
- **Periarticular osteopenia** – inflammation in the joint often causes reduction in bone mineral density, leading to darker areas adjacent to the articular surfaces on the X-ray.
- **Bone erosions** – synovial inflammation can invade and damage the cartilage and bony surfaces adjacent to the joint resulting in the development of bony erosions which may be visible on the X-ray. In RA, these are often referred to as 'marginal or juxta-articular bone erosions'.
- **Joint space narrowing** – damage to cartilage from persistent inflammation can lead to joint space narrowing. The joint space in RA is usually uniformly narrowed reflecting the generalised synovial inflammation affecting the whole joint.
- **Secondary signs** – as the condition progresses, there may be more extensive bone and cartilage destruction, remodelling, subluxation and dislocation and deformity may occur, for example ulnar deviation at the metacarpophalangeal (MCP) joints.

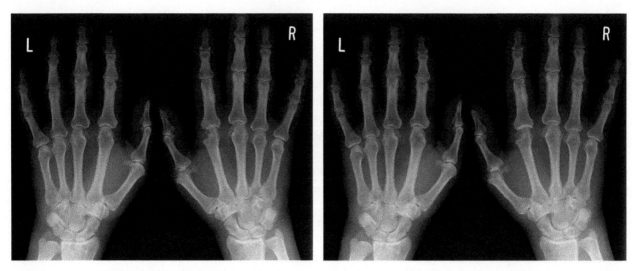

Figure 3.4 Rheumatoid arthritis. There are extensive erosions (orange) visible particularly in the metacarpal heads of the thumb, index and middle fingers on the right and middle finger on the left, together with scaphoid bone in the left wrist and ulnar styloid on the right seen *en face*. There is severe joint space narrowing in the right first and second MCP joints (green).

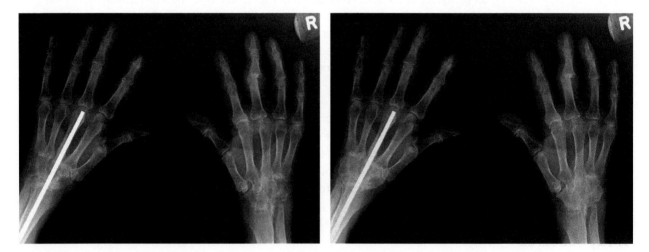

Figure 3.5 Severe established rheumatoid arthritis. There is evidence of a severe symmetrical destructive erosive polyarthropathy with almost complete fusion of the carpal joints bilaterally (green). The left wrist has been surgically fused. Further changes are seen more distally with periarticular osteopenia, erosive damage and deformity particularly affecting the right third MCP and proximal interphalangeal (PIP) joints where there is early subluxation.

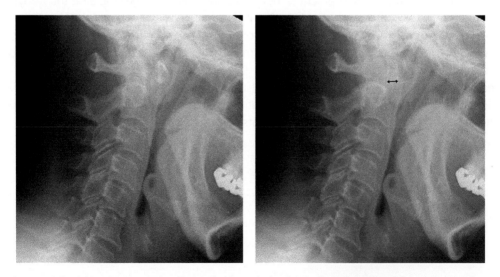

Figure 3.6 Atlanto-axial subluxation. Lateral radiograph of cervical spine in flexed position of a patient with established RA, demonstrating atlanto-axial subluxation with an anterior atlanto-dental interval of 7mm (yellow) (normal 2mm). This is measured (arrow) between the anterior arch of C1 (orange) and odontoid peg of C2 (green)

Crystal arthropathy

There is a range of arthropathies characterised by crystal deposition within joints and periarticular tissues which may be associated with acute self-limiting episodes of joint or soft tissue inflammation and chronic tissue damage.

The most common crystals and associated arthropathies include the following:
- Monosodium urate (MSU) – gout.
- Calcium pyrophosphate dihydrate (CPPD) – calcium pyrophosphate disease including asymptomatic chondrocalcinosis, acute pseudogout and a chronic destructive arthropathy.
- Basic calcium phosphate (hydroxyapatite) – calcific tendonitis, inflammatory exacerbations of OA, destructive arthropathy, for example Milwaukee shoulder.

Gout

Gout is the most common type of inflammatory arthritis in men. Gout occurs when crystals of uric acid, in the form of MSU, precipitate on the surface of articular cartilage, on tendons and in the surrounding tissues, provoking an inflammatory reaction. It most commonly occurs in patients who under-excrete urate due to kidney impairment or in those who overproduce urate, for example purine-rich diet or increased protein turnover in haematological diseases such as leukaemia or lymphoma.

The diagnosis is often made clinically, but demonstration of uric acid crystals by compensated polarised light microscopy examination of fluid aspirated from an affected joint enables a definitive diagnosis of gout by demonstration of needle-shaped, negatively birefringent MSU crystals. Joint fluid aspiration is important to exclude septic arthritis which may also present with an acutely hot, red and swollen joint.

Radiographs may be used as part of the diagnostic process or to monitor progression over time. In the acute setting the only visible sign may be soft tissue swelling but with repeated acute attacks, a number of characteristic radiographic features may develop.

Typical patient
A middle-aged or elderly man with a history of renal impairment, who may be overweight and taking diuretics, presents as an emergency with sudden onset of severely painful, hot, red, swollen big toe MTP joint, with a history of similar previous episodes.

Distribution

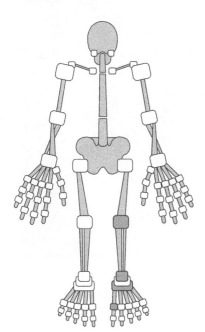

Gout is usually a monoarthritis most commonly affecting the great toe MTP joint. The midfoot, ankle and knee joints are the next most commonly affected and lower limb joint are more frequently involved than upper limb joints. It may also present as an oligoarthritis or polyarthritis.

Clinical practice points

Acute gout is characterised by excruciating, sudden, unexpected burning pain, as well as swelling, redness, warmth and stiffness in the affected joint, usually a monoarthritis of the great toe MTP joint (although an oligoarthritis, polyarthritis or chemical cellulitis may occur). Presentation may mimic septic arthritis.

Attacks often begin during the night and the patient wakes in great pain. These gout flares may resolve spontaneously, but often symptoms are so bad patients present as an emergency and require specific treatment with NSAIDs, colchicine or corticosteroids.

Recurrent attacks are common and can lead to joint damage and deformity as well as accumulation of uric acid deposits around joints called tophi. Treatment for recurrent gout involves managing modifiable risk factors and treating hyperuricaemia usually with medications such as allopurinol. The lower the serum uric acid, the less likely that there will be further attacks of acute gout.

> Gout is common, affecting 1–2 in 100 people in the UK, especially middle-aged men (most common form of inflammatory arthritis in males >40 years) with incidence increasing with age.
>
> Risk factors for gout can be divided into *non-modifiable* (e.g. age, sex, race, genetic factors and chronic kidney disease) and *modifiable* (e.g. hyperuricaemia, high-purine diet, consumption of purine-rich alcoholic beverages, obesity and certain medications particularly diuretics).

X-ray features

- **Soft tissue swelling** – soft tissue enlargement may be visible, reflecting generalised inflammation.
- **Bone erosions** – persistent inflammation will cause damage to the bone surface and the development of erosions which may be visible on X-ray. These erosions tend to occur just away from the joint margin and are described as 'para-articular' (in contrast to RA 'periarticular' erosions) and often look more spherical and deep with a punched-out appearance with sclerotic margins and overhanging edges.
- **Tophi** – may be visible as focal soft tissue densities which sometimes contain calcified deposits.
- **Secondary signs** – recurrent episodes may result in more extensive bone destruction with progression of erosions, joint space narrowing and deformity.

Note: Joint spaces are usually preserved unless severe and periarticular osteopenia is much less common.

(a)

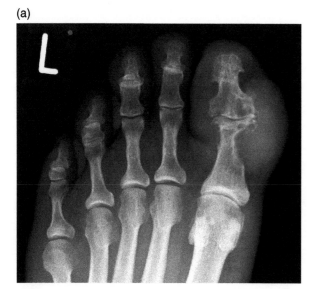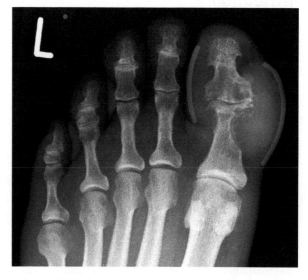

Figure 3.7 (a) Gout affecting left great toe. There is soft tissue swelling (yellow) and severe erosive changes (purple) which are characteristically wide based and 'punched out', located just away from the interphalangeal joint margin.

(b)

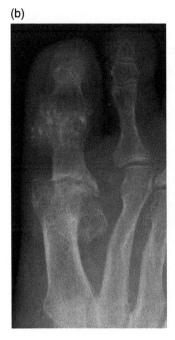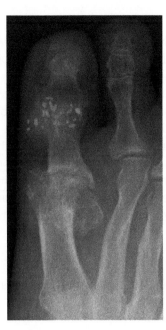

Figure 3.7 (b) Tophaceous gout great toe. There is a destructive arthropathy affecting the great toe MTP and interphalangeal (IP) joints, with severe erosive damage shown as loss of clarity of bone margins (orange), marked joint space loss (green), soft tissue swelling and tophaceous deposits in the soft tissues with punctate calcification (pink) adjacent to the IP joint.

Calcium pyrophosphate disease

Calcium pyrophosphate disease is common, especially in older people, and is characterised by deposition of CPPD crystals predominantly in articular hyaline and fibrocartilage (chondrocalcinosis).

A variety of clinical manifestations may occur including the following:

- asymptomatic incidental finding of chondrocalcinosis
- acute inflammatory mono- or oligoarthritis (acute CPP arthritis or 'pseudo-gout'), which is the most common cause of monoarthritis in the elderly
- chronic asymmetric destructive arthritis – OA plus CPPD (previously termed chronic pyrophosphate arthropathy)

Diagnosis is usually made in the presence of a characteristic clinical presentation supported by identification of typical crystals (non-birefringent or weakly positively birefringent rods or rhomboids) on compensated polarised light microscopy of synovial fluid. Radiographs can be useful to demonstrate calcification and any bone and cartilage destruction that may develop over time, and often help in making the diagnosis.

Typical patient

An elderly woman, with a history of OA, presents with acute inflammatory monoarthritis of the knee, perhaps precipitated by intercurrent illness or infection, or surgery.

Distribution

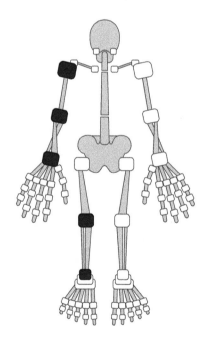

Acute 'pseudogout' is typically a monoarthritis most commonly affecting the knee, then wrist, shoulder ankle and elbow joints.

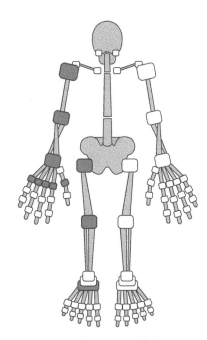

Chronic pyrophosphate arthropathy is usually an oligoarthritis, most commonly affecting the knee, then wrist, shoulder, elbow, hip, midtarsal and MCP joints. It may also present as a monoarthritis or polyarthritis. Note overlap with OA.

Clinical practice points

Acute pseudogout usually presents as an inflammatory monoarthritis, with sudden onset of severe pain, stiffness and swelling. There are clinical signs of synovitis including joint effusion, tenderness, redness, warmth and restricted movement. Fever is common and elderly patients may become generally unwell and confused. Presentation may mimic septic arthritis.

Chronic pyrophosphate arthropathy is usually an oligoarticular pattern and overlaps with OA, with more chronic joint symptoms including pain, early morning and inactivity stiffness, reduced movement and functional impairment, superimposed by acute pseudogout episodes.

Effective anti-inflammatory treatment, particularly for acute episodes, is available, using NSAIDs, corticosteroids or colchicine, but treating chronic forms is more challenging.

> Chondrocalcinosis may be present in up to one-third of healthy people aged 65–75.
> Familial and sporadic forms may occur.
> It may be associated with metabolic disease, for example primary hyperparathyroidism and haemochromatosis.

X-ray features

- Cartilage and soft tissue calcification
  - Chondrocalcinosis
    - Fibrocartilage, for example knee menisci, wrist triangular fibrocartilage and symphysis pubis
    - Hyaline cartilage, for example knee, glenohumeral joint (GHJ) and hip
  - Capsular and synovial calcification, for example MCPs and knee
  - Entheseal calcification, for example Achilles, triceps and obturator tendons
  - Bursal calcification, for example subacromial, olecranon and retrocalcaneal

Soft tissue deposits have a calcific density but no structure. They can be distinguished from ossification or a bony fragment as they lack trabeculation or a cortex. These may disappear after the acute inflammatory episode has settled and the crystals have been resorbed and so may not be visible on subsequent X-rays.

- OA changes may predominate, that is *cartilage loss, subchondral sclerosis and cysts and osteophytes*
- Features particular to CPPD contributing to 'hypertrophic' appearance and distribution include the following:
  - Involvement of joints less typical of OA, for example MCPs, GHJ, ankle, radio-carpal joint (RCJ) associated with scaphoid–lunate dissociation and midfoot.
  - Prominent *'exuberant' osteophytes* and *large subchondral cysts* (especially knee and wrist).
  - Smooth *'pressure' erosions* may occur, for example anterior distal femur, distal inferior radio-ulna and radiocarpal joints.
- The relatively rare variant of destructive pyrophosphate arthropathy may cause marked *cartilage and bone loss* with changes eventually resembling a Charcot joint.

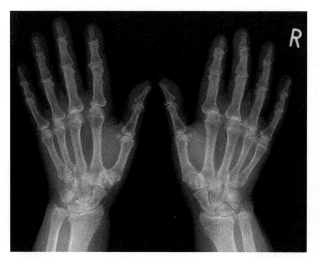 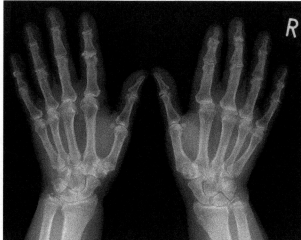

Figure 3.8 Calcium pyrophosphate arthropathy of the hands and wrists. There is chondrocalcinosis in the triangular fibrocartilage at the ulna–carpal compartments of both wrists (pink), joint space loss (green) and osteophyte formation at the MCPs (purple) and a background of changes of osteoarthritis affecting a number of PIP, DIP and first carpometacarpal (CMC) joints (blue).

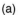

(a)

(b)

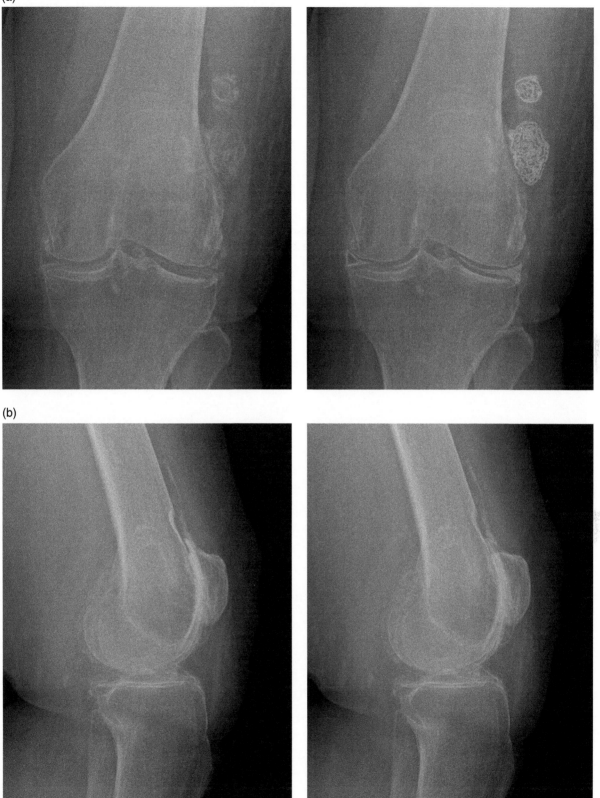

Figure 3.9 Calcium pyrophosphate arthropathy of the knee. (a) Anterior view and (b) lateral view. There are typical features of calcium pyrophosphate arthropathy with chondrocalcinosis at the tibiofemoral joints (pink), severe secondary degenerative changes at the patellofemoral joint with marked joint space loss (green), subchondral sclerosis (blue) and osteophytes (purple) and scalloping at the anterior distal femur consistent with a 'pressure erosion' (orange). There is further calcification of the synovium in the suprapatellar pouch and also some ossified bodies projected in the lateral recess of the suprapatellar pouch and popliteal fossa (yellow).

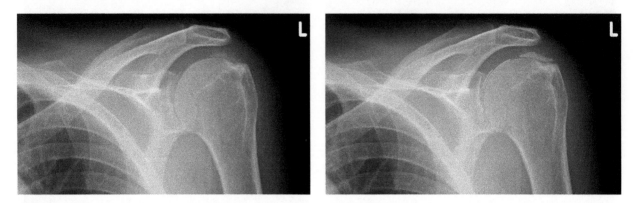

Figure 3.10 Prominent chondrocalcinosis (blue) and amorphous calcification in the region of supraspinatus tendon (yellow). The appearances are of calcium deposition disease within the joint and tendon.

Psoriatic arthritis

Psoriatic arthritis (PsA) is a chronic inflammatory arthropathy which can affect up to 20% of patients with skin or nail psoriasis. Psoriasis is an inflammatory skin disease characterised by red scaly plaques usually affecting the extensor surfaces of elbows and knees, hairline and umbilicus. In some patients with PsA, there may be a family history of psoriasis and skin psoriasis may not necessarily be apparent. There is a genetic link to HLA-B27, so other conditions such as inflammatory bowel or eye disease may also be associated. It is considered a type of seronegative spondyloarthritis and can cause arthritis, enthesitis, tensosynovitis, dactylitis and spondylitis.

X-rays are important in the assessment of patients with PsA, but like the clinical manifestations, a variety of different changes and inconsistent manifestations may be seen in a range of sites including peripheral synovial joints, axial skeleton and fibrocartilagenous joints (e.g. sacroiliac joint) as well as entheseal attachments of ligaments and tendons.

Typical patient
A middle-aged patient (30–55 years) with a history of skin psoriasis and nail pitting and a previous episode of uveitis, presents with pain, stiffness and swelling affecting the left knee and several different finger joints in an asymmetrical distribution.

Distribution
There is considerable variety in the pattern of joint involvement but asymmetry is common. Patients are traditionally classified into one of the following five sub-types:
1. Predominant DIP finger joints involvement (Figure 1)
2. Asymmetrical mono- or oligoarthritis, usually knees and small peripheral joints (Figure 2)
3. Symmetrical polyarthritis (like RA) (Figure 3)
4. Spondyloarthritis (spine and sacroiliac joints) (Figure 4)
5. Arthritis mutilans with destruction, osteolysis and telescoping of the fingers (Figure 5)

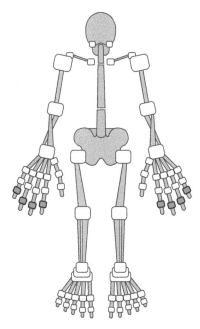

Figure 1

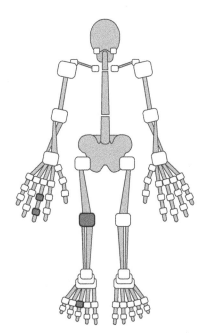

Figure 2

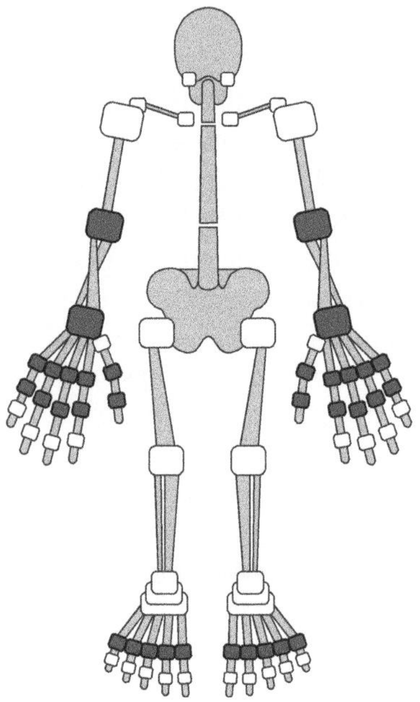

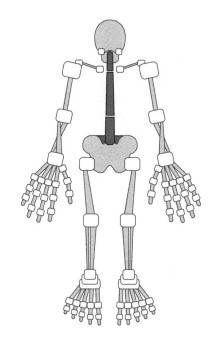

Figure 3

Figure 4

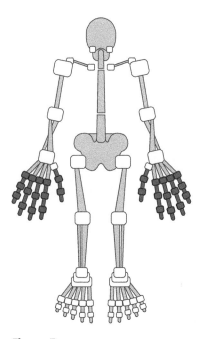

Figure 5

Clinical practice points

Like RA, radiographic findings may be absent, especially in early disease. Extra-articular manifestations associated with the *HLA-B27* gene may occur, particularly inflammatory eye disease, for example anterior uveitis.

Up to a quarter of patients with PsA may have sacroiliitis, and changes may be more extensive and are more likely to be asymmetrical than in axial spondyloarthritis (aSpA) (ankylosing spondylitis). Treatments include NSAIDs, glucocorticoids, disease-modifying anti-rheumatic drugs (DMARDs), for example methotrexate or biologic therapies, for example tumour necrosis factor (TNF)-alpha inhibitors.

> There may not be a direct association between the severity of skin and joint disease.
> The characteristic radiological hallmark of PsA is a combination of bone destruction and new bone formation.
> Angulated views of the sacroiliac joint (e.g. modified Ferguson view) may help improve sensitivity.
> Grading systems can be applied to quantify the severity of sacroiliitis but MRI is the best imaging method to demonstrate sacroiliitis.

X-ray features

- **Soft tissue swelling** – may be caused by joint, tendon or soft tissue swelling and dactylitis.
- **Erosions** – usually well-defined and situated in a periarticular location (similar to RA) but are more likely to be asymmetric.
- **Proliferative new bone formation** – characteristic and often coexists with erosive changes sometimes giving an ill-defined spiculated appearance at the joint margin.
- **Joint space narrowing** – may develop as the disease progresses.
- **Periostitis** – inflammation of periosteal surface particularly at the shaft may be visible as increased radiographic density adjacent to the bony surface.
- **Sacroiliitis** – erosions and new bone formation may occur in the sacroiliac joints producing irregular margins and sclerosis, making these joints difficult to clearly delineate on the X-ray.
- **Spondylitis** – may be visible as bony proliferation (syndesmophytes) throughout the spine, but bridging between vertebra is less common.
- **Bony proliferation at entheseal attachments** – for example at the insertions of the Achilles tendon and plantar fascia to the calcaneum and entheseal sites around the pelvis.
- **'Pencil in cup' deformity, osteolysis and ankylosis** – progressive bone destruction and osteolysis particularly in the finger end joints may result in a pointed appearance of the phalanx tip and a pronounced curved appearance caused by new bone formation at the base of the adjacent phalanx, giving a 'pencil in cup' appearance.

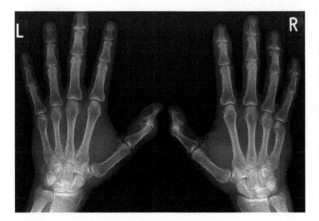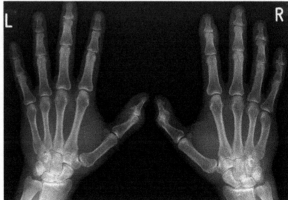

Figure 3.11 Psoriatic arthritis finger DIP joints. A combination of erosions (orange) and new bone formation (purple) affecting the DIP joints of left thumb and middle finger and right thumb and all fingers, at different stages of severity.

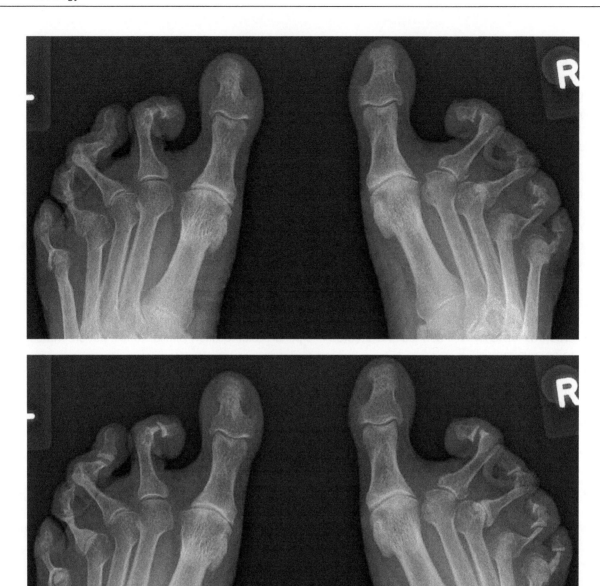

Figure 3.12 Psoriatic arthritis feet. Severe psoriatic arthropathy and deformity of the distal toes with erosions, osteolysis and some new bone formation and 'pencil in cup' deformities at a number of MTP and IP joints (yellow).

Axial spondyloarthritis (ankylosing spondylitis)

Axial Spondyloarthritis (aSpA) (ankylosing spondylitis) is characterised by inflammation affecting the sacroiliac joints and spine. Like PsA, it is strongly associated with *HLA-B27* and so shares a number of similar clinical features, disease associations and familial predominance.

Patients are usually young (typically males aged 15-35 years) and present with persistent pain and stiffness affecting the lower back region. Unfortunately, the diagnosis is often delayed with a long lag time between symptom onset and formal diagnosis and often patients have sought medical attention or just coped with their symptoms a long time before a formal diagnosis is made, perhaps because back pain is common and usually mechanical in origin.

The diagnosis relies on a combination of clinical and imaging criteria, and newer guidelines allow the use of MRI in addition to X-rays, which improves their sensitivity. The first radiographic sign is usually symmetrical sacroiliitis, which is highly specific for this condition, but this often takes a long time to develop (sometimes up to 9 years), and initial radiographs are often normal. Radiographic spondylitis may also be evident in the spine as well as ligamentous calcification.

Typical patient

A young man who has had back pain for almost 2 years which wakes him during the night and early morning. He has to take regular ibuprofen to gain some relief from his symptoms. His back is stiff with reduced lumbar lordosis and lateral spinal flexion. He is positive for *HLA-B27*.

Distribution

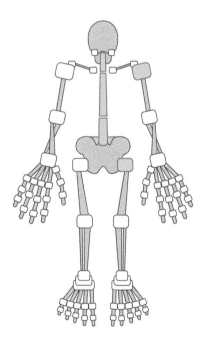

aSpA always involves the axial skeleton (sacroiliac joints and spine). There may also be asymmetrical involvement of the medium and large joints particularly shoulders and hips. Inflammation at sites of bony insertion of tendons and ligaments (enthesitis) is common at sites including iliac crests, gluteal and tibial tuberosities and heels.

Clinical practice points

The diagnostic and classification criteria have evolved over time, and most authors often now refer to this spectrum of diseases as spondyloarthritis (SpA), subdivided into axial SpA (aSpA) (which is further divided into classical ankylosing spondylitis and non-radiographic aSpA) and predominantly peripheral SpA (which includes PsA, reactive arthritis, arthritis with inflammatory bowel disease and undifferentiated SpA).

Treatments include NSAIDs, glucocorticoids, DMARDs (e.g. sulphasalazine) or biologic therapies (e.g. TNF-alpha inhibitors).

Back pain is common in the general population and only approximately 5% will have aSpA.

HLA-B27 is also a common gene present in approximately 8% of the Caucasian population, but only 1 in 4 of these will develop aSpA. Up to 90% of patients with aSpA are *HLA-B27*-positive, and this gene is a marker for more severe disease. However, it is important to note racial differences in *HLA B27* prevalence.

The diagnosis of aSpA is often delayed by up to 6–8 years, often because X-rays are normal in the early stages of the disease.

MRI is much more sensitive than X-rays at detecting the early signs of aSpA as it can detect both inflammation (bone marrow oedema) and structural changes (erosions).

X-ray features

- **Sacroiliitis** – usually bilateral and symmetrical, affecting the lower third (synovial part), particularly the iliac side of the joint. There may be loss of clarity of the joint margins, erosions, joint space widening with subsequent bony proliferation and sclerosis. As the changes progress, the joint space margins will become more indistinct and will gradually disappear as ankylosis eventually develops.
- **Spondylitis** – erosions and new bone formation occur at the corners of vertebral bodies usually beginning in the thoracolumbar junction, forming 'Romanus lesions'. New bone will then form along the anterior aspect of the vertebral body reversing the normal concavity producing a squared appearance. Calcification occurs in the adjacent intervertebral disc and longitudinal spinal ligaments forming syndesmophytes which may proliferate forming bony spurs and join with similar lesions from adjacent vertebra leading to a characteristic 'bamboo spine' appearance of established aSpA and eventually ankylosis.
- **Soft tissue calcification** – ligamentous calcification may occur, for example in the posterior ligamentous portion of the sacroiliac joint and the posterior interspinous ligament.
- **Bone density** – may be generally reduced.

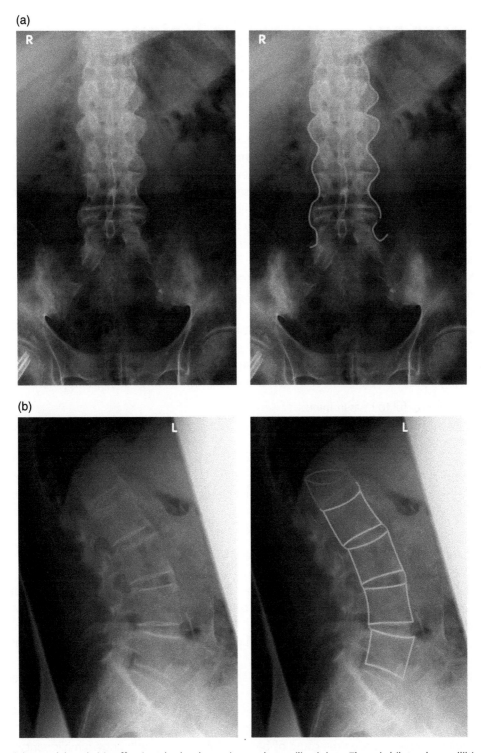

Figure 3.13 Axial spondyloarthritis affecting the lumbar spine and sacroiliac joints. There is bilateral sacroiliitis and fusion of the sacroiliac joints (yellow), squaring of the vertebral bodies (blue), bridging syndesmophytes with a 'bamboo spine' appearance in the thoracolumbar spine (pink), an anterior wedge fracture (purple) likely to be related to low bone density, and screws are just visible in the right femoral head from internal fixation of a previous fractured neck of femur (orange).

4 Tumours and tumour-like lesions

This chapter discusses benign and malignant tumours as well as tumour-like lesions occurring in the skeleton. Rather than attempting to include the large range of tumours which exist, the intention is to explain the important principles and describe a logical approach to evaluation, whilst illustrating the most important lesions in more detail. The term 'tumour-like lesion' is used for an abnormality which may look similar to a tumour on X-rays but is not a neoplasm, for example a fibrous cortical defect or an area of osteomyelitis.

Many focal bone lesions have relatively specific X-ray features which help to narrow down the likely diagnosis, but the principle that X-ray findings are never considered in isolation is once again very important. The whole clinical context must be taken into account. Factors including the patient's age, previous medical history, current symptoms and blood and other laboratory test results are all essential clues to the diagnosis. It is also extremely important to find out whether there is a single bone lesion or several, as this alters the likely diagnosis.

Many bone lesions occur at typical sites and in specific age groups, so it is essential to also take these factors into account.

Once the X-ray findings, along with the aforementioned information, have been gathered it is possible to suggest either a single probable diagnosis or a differential diagnosis of three or so possibilities.

Some basic facts are useful to bear in mind:
- Malignant primary bone tumours are rare, so it is likely that one will only be seen every few years in an orthopaedic clinic.
- The diagnosis of a malignant primary bone tumour should be considered in any child or young adult with bone pain and/or a mass.
- Over the age of 40, metastases and myeloma should be the first consideration when a patient presents with a suspected malignant bone lesion.

Radiological evaluation of the patient

Setting aside the clinical information, blood and any other laboratory results for the time being, the radiological evaluation of a patient who might have a bone tumour can be tackled in terms of first detecting whether a bony abnormality is present and, if so, characterising it.

Primary malignant bone tumours tend to be visible on plain X-rays when the patient presents, as do most benign bone tumours.

X-rays are less sensitive for metastases and myeloma, so the detection or exclusion requires other imaging modalities.

MRI is highly sensitive for detecting focal abnormalities in bone and can readily demonstrate lesions as small as 5 mm. It is most commonly used to evaluate a specific symptomatic area rather than the whole skeleton. Common indications include assessing the cause of back pain in patients with known malignancy; investigating suspected cord compression from spinal metastatic disease, as the cord and nerve roots are also visualised (Figure 4.1); and also for staging multiple myeloma. MRI has the advantage of directly imaging the bone marrow tissue. X-rays are excellent for showing changes in the calcified structural elements of the bone but metastases, myeloma and also bone lymphoma are shown with greater sensitivity by MRI because they initially

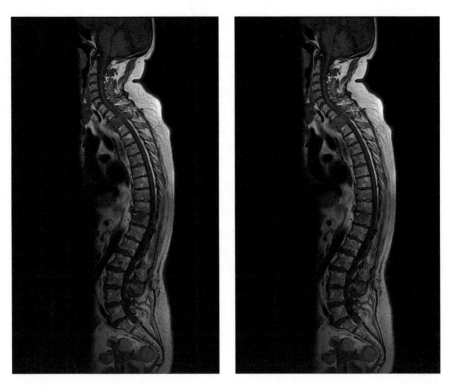

Figure 4.1 MRI of the spine (T1-weighted sequence) in a patient with vertebral metastases at T2, T11 and L2 (red). The tumour shows as low-signal (dark) deposits against the high-signal fat of normal bone marrow. The T2 lesion extends into the vertebral canal producing early compression of the spinal cord.

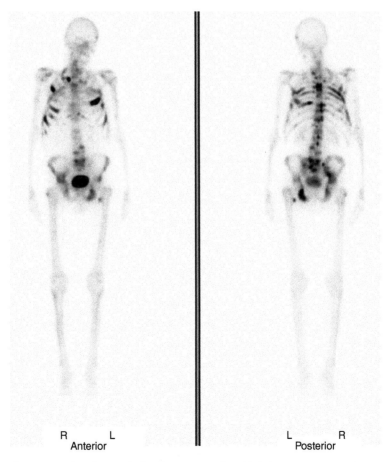

R L
Anterior

L R
Posterior

Figure 4.2 Radioisotope bone scan showing typical appearances of multiple bone metastases in a patient with prostate cancer. Increased isotope activity due to metastases shows as dark areas on the image. The deposits have a predisposition for the axial skeleton, and within this area they are randomly scattered and of various sizes.

infiltrate and replace the normal marrow before any visible changes develop in the calcified structural tissues of bone. Bone marrow oedema is also shown well by MRI, allowing better detection of lesions which are associated with this, such as occult fractures, osteomyelitis and osteoid osteoma.

A radioisotope bone scan (aka bone scintigraphy) is commonly used to investigate suspected metastatic disease. It is also a sensitive imaging test which can show bone lesions before they become visible on X-ray (Figure 4.2). A bone-seeking agent (such as hydroxymethylene diphosphonate – HDP) with an attached gamma radiation–emitting marker technetium 99m is injected into a peripheral vein. Four hours after the injection, a gamma camera can be used to image the whole skeleton. An anterior and a posterior view are obtained. Nearly all types of bone metastases are demonstrated as focal areas of increased isotope activity, or 'hot spots'. However, other pathological processes, such as fractures and arthropathy, will also produce increased activity on a bone scan and therefore the distribution of lesions, the clinical situation and sometimes the appearances on other imaging studies all need to be considered in its interpretation. Although an isotope bone scan is a sensitive test for nearly all metastatic disease, it is poor at detecting myeloma/plasmacytoma and purely lytic metastases.

X-rays – general principles

Plain X-rays are of vital importance when it comes to assessing the nature of a focal bone lesion. The clues or signs on the X-ray help considerably in determining the probable diagnosis and also for excluding other diagnoses.

Location is important, both in terms of which area of the skeleton is involved, and also the specific site within a given bone. Many tumours and other focal lesions are commonly found at certain sites. For example, the majority of osteosarcomas occur in the long bone metaphyses, particularly in the proximal humerus or on either side of the knee joint.

From clues ('radiological signs') on an X-ray, it may be possible to tell whether a lesion is aggressive or relatively benign. Bone reacts differently to rapidly and slowly growing lesions, and these changes are better shown on plain films than MRI or other modalities.

The pattern of calcification within a lesion can be characteristic, for example the 'popcorn' appearance of cartilaginous lesions (Figure 4.3).

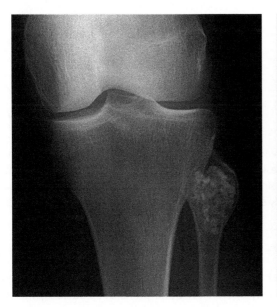 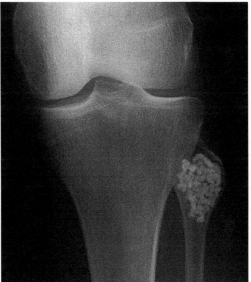

Figure 4.3 An enchondroma in the fibular head found incidentally on an X-ray taken for a knee injury. The characteristic pattern of calcification in cartilaginous lesions resembles popcorn.

Also bone changes around the margins of the lesion are important.

We can think about the margins of a lesion in two areas: (1) outward extension, as the lesion encounters cortex and may extend through the periosteum and into the soft tissues and (2) extension within the trabecular bone, usually along the medullary cavity of a long bone. The bony response to the lesion differs depending on whether it is *aggressive or slow-growing*. Aggressive lesions spread both along the bone inside the medullary cavity and sideways through the cortex at a rate which does not allow the surrounding bone to lay down a clearly defined margin. Each time the bone's response begins, the lesion advances before the changes can be completed. This means that as a fast-growing lesion spreads along the medullary cavity the bone texture may alter on the X-ray but it is unclear where the abnormality ends and the normal bone begins (Figures 4.4a and 4.5a). On the other hand, a slowly growing lesion is demarcated from the surrounding bone by a sharp, clear and often sclerotic, edge with a normal trabecular pattern beyond because the native bone has had time to adapt (Figures 4.4b and 4.5b). Therefore, the width of this zone between definitely abnormal and definitely normal bone texture directly reflects the speed with which the lesion is infiltrating along the medullary cavity.

In terms of lateral spread at or beyond the cortex, pathology which is aggressive may cause areas of cortical destruction, seen as interruption of the white line of the cortex (Figure 4.5a), while less aggressive

(a)

(b)

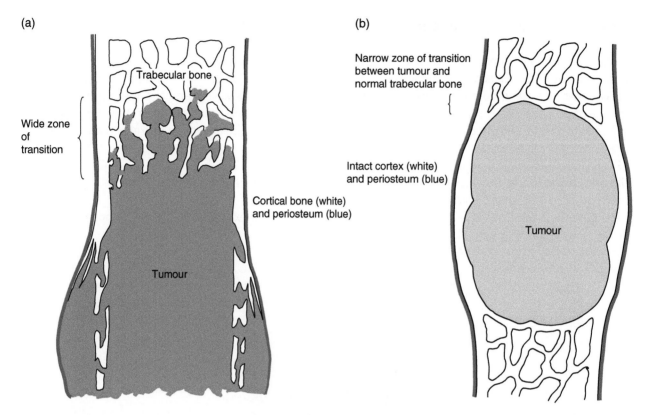

Figure 4.4 A tumour will extend along the medullary cavity, where it encounters trabecular bone, and 'sideways', where it encounters the cortex and periosteum. (a) A fast-growing lesion moves through the medullary cavity and cortex before the bone can react to form a clear line of demarcation. (b) A slow-growing tumour enlarges at a rate which allows the trabecular bone to form a clearer margin, and may also slowly erode the endosteal surface of the cortex, while allowing mature periosteal new bone to develop on the outer aspect.

lesions leave the cortex intact. Once through the cortex, aggressive lesions elevate the periosteum and infiltrate through it. As the role of the periosteum is to lay down new bone on its deep surface, this will begin to happen. However, as the lesion is constantly enlarging, the process cannot be completed. Therefore, aggressive lesions are associated with irregular, incomplete periosteal changes. Periosteal new bone has the best chance to form near the margin of the elevated area, producing what is known as a 'Codman triangle' (Figure 4.6a). On the other hand, a slow-growing lesion may induce periosteal new bone formation but it has a clear and smooth appearance reflecting the time it has had to develop in an organised way (Figure 4.6b).

Again remember to look for soft tissue swelling, which often reflects an aggressive tumour but may also occur with osteomyelitis or a pathological fracture.

Although aggressive (i.e. rapidly enlarging) lesions are often malignant, they are not invariably so as, for example, osteomyelitis may also produce aggressive changes in bone. Also some slowly growing lesions may be malignant.

By combining all the clues, particularly the clinical background, patient's age, exact location(s) and X-ray features, it is possible to narrow down the differential diagnosis of bone lesions. This then allows decisions to be made concerning further management, for example biopsy of a suspected metastasis or referral to a regional bone tumour service for a suspected primary malignant bone tumour. It is not always possible to make a specific diagnosis, but the overall findings certainly help to determine a shorter differential and therefore guide what steps should be taken next.

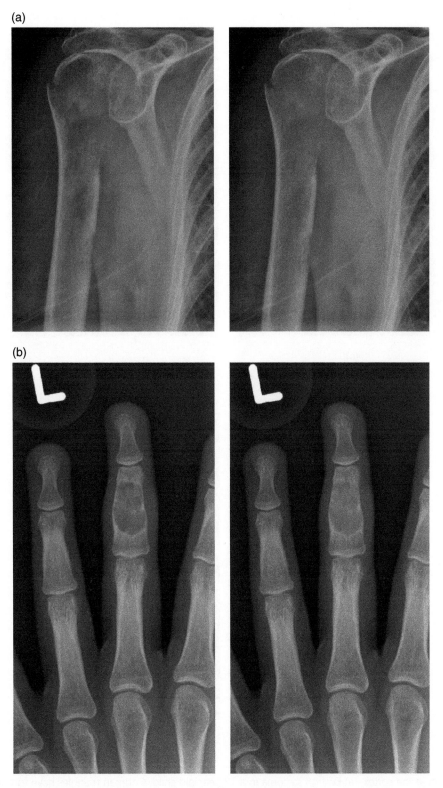

Figure 4.5 Extension in the medullary cavity: At the margin of an aggressive lesion such as this lung cancer metastasis (a), it is difficult to determine exactly where abnormal bone ends and normal trabecular bone begins (*a wide zone of transition*). There is also a pathological fracture passing obliquely through the surgical neck of the humerus, shown by disruption of the medial and lateral cortices at the level of the lytic lesion. By contrast, a slowly growing benign enchondroma (b) shows a clear demarcation where it abuts normal trabecular bone (*narrow zone of transition*).

(a)

(b)

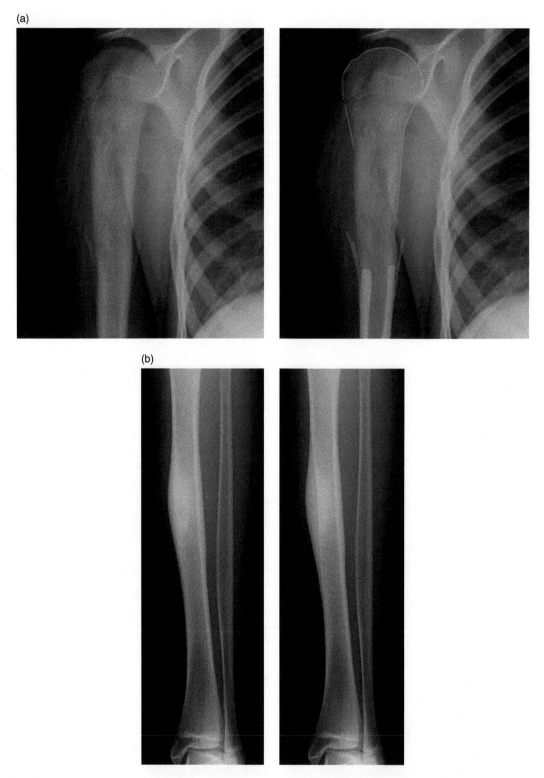

Figure 4.6 Extension at the cortex: (a) Ewing's sarcoma in a 12-year-old child. Codman triangles have formed at the margins of the elevated periosteum (green). Rapid extension of tumour into the surrounding soft tissues has also resulted in loss of definition of the white line of the cortex (normal cortex in yellow). There is a wide zone of transition within the medullary cavity. (b) Osteoid osteoma in the mid-shaft of the tibia. The periosteal bone formation provoked by this benign lesion has a smooth, well-defined appearance reflecting its non-aggressive nature and lack of extension through the cortex.

Malignant tumours

Metastases and multiple myeloma are by far the most common types of malignant tumour found in the bone. Plasmacytoma is not uncommon, but other primary malignant bone tumours such as osteosarcoma, chondrosarcoma and Ewing's sarcoma are in fact rare (bone sarcomas account for 0.2% of new cancers per year). For example, a GP might only see one or two patients with these primary tumours during their career compared with large numbers of patients with bone metastases and myeloma.

Bone metastases

Metastases are by far the most common neoplasm found in bone. Although virtually any primary cancer can metastasise to the skeleton, the tumours which have the highest tendency to do so are prostate, breast, lung, renal and thyroid. These account for about 80% of metastases in adults. In children, neuroblastoma is the most common cause of bone metastases.

Blood-borne metastases tend to spread through the venous system. The axial skeleton (skull, spine, ribs, scapulae, pelvis and proximal femora and humeri) and also liver and lungs are all common sites for metastases to develop. In the case of the latter two, this is believed to be because of their role as venous filters. The preponderance of bone metastases is thought to relate to other factors: a network of paraspinal veins has tributaries from the abdomen, pelvis, thorax and upper and lower limbs which allow access to the bones of the axial skeleton, bypassing the normal filters of the liver and lungs. The primary purpose of the bone marrow in these areas is haematopoiesis, and the vascular permeability intended for access of these cells into the bloodstream from the marrow also allows malignant cells to pass in the opposite direction. The nutrient-rich environment intended for erythropoiesis enables the metastatic cells to multiply.

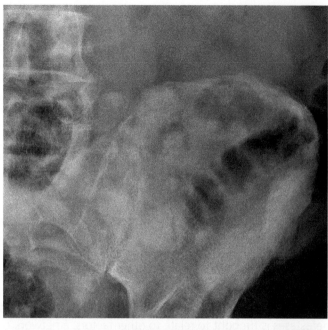

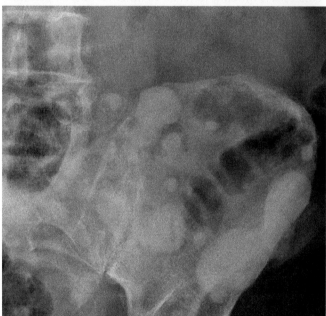

Figure 4.7 Sclerotic bone metastases in the pelvis of an 80-year-old man with carcinoma of the prostate, visible as increased density compared with normal bone. The lesions are multiple, of varying size and located in the axial skeleton. (The areas of lucency are due to bowel gas projected over the bone.)

Bone metastases are rare in the peripheral skeleton. Those that do occur are usually from a lung primary and are believed to spread via the arterial system. The primary tumour invades a pulmonary vein, passes through the heart and subsequently ends up in the systemic arterial circulation.

X-ray features

Multiplicity is the characteristic feature of metastases. Other features are variable. Generally, metastases do not have sufficiently specific features to diagnose what the primary will be. The plain film appearances can vary from lytic (Figure 4.5a), sclerotic (Figure 4.7) or a mixture of the two. They may be well defined or show a poorly demarcated pattern. Soft tissue extension beyond the bone and its associated periosteal reaction is uncommon with metastatic disease. Expansion of the cortex may sometimes occur, most typically with renal and thyroid metastases.

It is also important to be aware that despite the presence of metastatic disease in the bone, plain X-rays will commonly not show any abnormality. In other words, a normal X-ray does not exclude the diagnosis.

Multiple myeloma

In a patient over 40 years of age with multiple bone lesions, it is useful to think of both myeloma and metastatic disease as likely causes.

Myeloma is the most common primary malignant tumour occurring in bone. It is a malignancy of plasma cells which arises in the marrow, but as disease progresses the structural calcified elements of the bones also become involved. The clonally duplicated plasma cells usually secrete paraprotein (most often IgG), and this can be detected in the blood for diagnostic purposes by plasma electrophoresis or in the urine as Bence Jones protein. They may also secrete substances which suppress osteoblastic and promote osteoclastic activity resulting in secondary osteoporosis. Associated insufficiency fractures may lead to the first presentation.

Seventy-five per cent of patients are over the age of 50 years, with a peak between 60 and 70 years. Myeloma is very rare in those under 40 years.

Because it is a disease of active bone marrow, its distribution is primarily within the axial skeleton.

X-ray features
The appearance of multiple myeloma deposits has been likened to raindrops on a dry pavement. The lesions are multiple, lytic and have a well-defined, punched-out appearance (Figure 4.8). In advanced disease, the bone texture develops a more generalised coarse appearance (Figure 4.9).

Myeloma is usually undetectable on a nuclear medicine bone scan due to a lack of osteoblastic activity. However, MRI is sensitive at revealing deposits due to their altered signal compared to surrounding normal fatty adult marrow. As a result, MRI of the spine, a common site of involvement, is used for staging the disease. It will reveal abnormalities which are not shown on an X-ray skeletal survey.

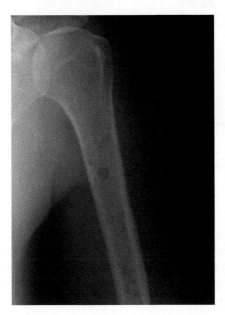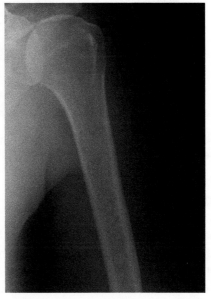

Figure 4.8 Multiple myeloma in a 72-year-old woman. There are multiple, small, well-defined, lytic tumours 'splashed' along the humeral shaft. Multiple myeloma typically involves the axial skeleton initially but is more easily visible when it involves the long bones or skull.

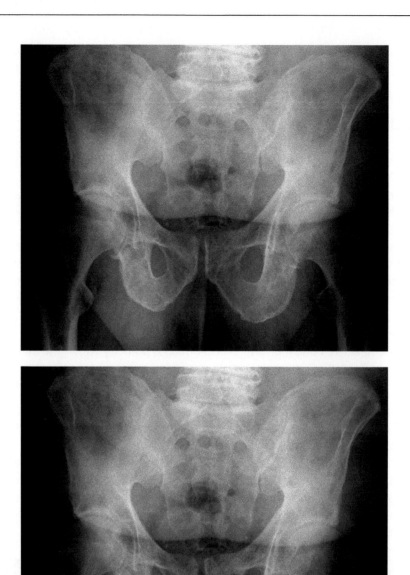

Figure 4.9 Multiple myeloma. Bone involvement is less clearly visible in the axial skeleton on X-rays, but there is subtle alteration of texture in the left ischiopubic ramus, with a coarsened appearance of the trabecular bone.

Plasmacytoma

Multiple myeloma by definition involves multiple sites. A focal solitary lesion consisting of the same pathology is referred to as a plasmacytoma. A patient with a plasmacytoma may develop multiple myeloma over time. On average, plasmacytoma may be found at an earlier age than myeloma, but patients still tend to be above 40 years. Protein electrophoresis is often normal. Tumours are found at sites of red marrow, that is in the axial skeleton.

X-ray features

Plasmacytoma typically has a purely lytic appearance. It may be expansile, producing endosteal thinning of the cortex (Figure 4.10). It shows features of a relatively slow growth rate with a narrow zone of transition. The differential is an expansile metastasis such as from a thyroid, breast or renal primary.

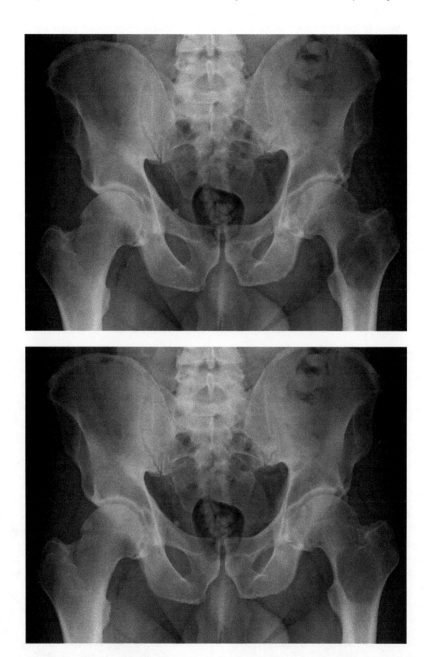

Figure 4.10 Plasmacytoma in a 60-year-old man. The tumour is purely lytic and centred in the medullary cavity of the proximal left femur. Although the tumour is malignant, the narrow zone of transition and lack of extension through the cortex reflect relatively slow growth.

Osteosarcoma

This is a tumour characterised by malignant osteoid-producing cells, resulting in areas of visible disorganised calcification within the tumour on X-rays.

Typically, the patient presents with pain and swelling. There is sometimes a coincidental history of trauma, which may initially be taken to be the cause of symptoms. Some patients present with a pathological fracture through the tumour site.

The peak age for presentation is 10–15 years. Osteosarcoma may also arise secondary to either previous radiotherapy or Paget's disease in older patients.

Osteosarcomas favour the metaphysis of a long bone, and 75% occur around the knee with the proximal humerus being another common site.

X-ray features

Osteosarcomas are usually relatively advanced at presentation, with established X-ray appearances (Figure 4.11). A typical tumour arises in the metaphysis, and is centred in the medullary cavity but extends through the cortex, forming a mass in the adjacent soft tissues. The mass may be visible beyond the cortex of the bone due to outward displacement of the adjacent soft tissue fat planes or calcification within the tumour matrix. There is aggressive periosteal reaction shown as a laminated or a 'sunburst' appearance with Codman triangles at the margins of the affected length of cortex. The zone of transition between obvious tumour and normal bone texture is wide.

The appearance within the tumour largely depends on the amount of bone being produced. It may be sclerotic or osteolytic only but usually has areas of both.

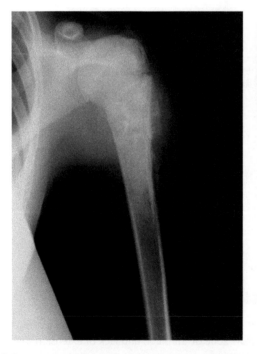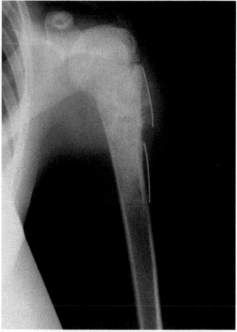

Figure 4.11 Osteosarcoma in the proximal humerus of a 13-year-old child. The lesion exhibits typical aggressive features of a malignant tumour with a wide zone of transition in the medullary cavity; irregular partial destruction of cortical bone and incomplete periosteal bone formation (green). The tumour has a mixed sclerotic and lytic appearance.

Chondrosarcoma

Chondrosarcoma is a malignant tumour of cartilage (chondroid) cells. There are two groups of chondrosarcoma. The first group comprises 90% of tumours which occur de novo within the medullary bone. The second group result from malignant transformation within a previously benign cartilage tumour, either an osteochondroma (exostosis) or an enchondroma (see below). For this reason, increased growth or pain in any chondroid lesion in an adult should be regarded as suspicious and prompt further evaluation.

De novo tumours tend to affect an older age group, most commonly in the sixth decade. Their behaviour and X-ray appearance vary depending on whether the tumour is well or poorly differentiated, but most typically the tumour is slow growing. There may be a history of insidious pain going back for several months or even years. Chondrosarcomas favour sites in the axial skeleton, especially the pelvis, proximal femur and proximal humerus.

X-ray features

The most common appearance is of a large, lucent lesion centred in the medullary cavity with a relatively narrow zone of transition (Figure 4.12a). The matrix may include areas of typical 'popcorn' chondroid calcification. However, this is not always the case and alternatively there may be areas of amorphous calcification or the lesion may be purely lucent. The endosteal surface of the surrounding cortex undergoes resorption due to pressure from the enlarging tumour. The appearance is referred to as endosteal scalloping and reflects the lobulated shape of the tumour. Meanwhile, periosteal thickening, with a relatively smooth and uninterrupted surface, reflecting slow growth, develops on the outside. Therefore, over time, the cortex develops a bulging appearance referred to as bony expansion. Less typically the tumour is aggressive with a wide zone of transition, cortical destruction and extension beyond the cortex.

Malignant transformation in an enchondroma will show similar X-ray features to those described above. In the early stages of transformation comparison with previous X-rays is very helpful to see if the lesion is enlarging Figure 4.12b. In the case of an exostosis the cartilage cap initially thickens. This is not visible on X-rays but can be shown with MRI, which should be performed if there is clinical suspicion. Later the bony component of the osteochondroma may show altered bone texture or destruction.

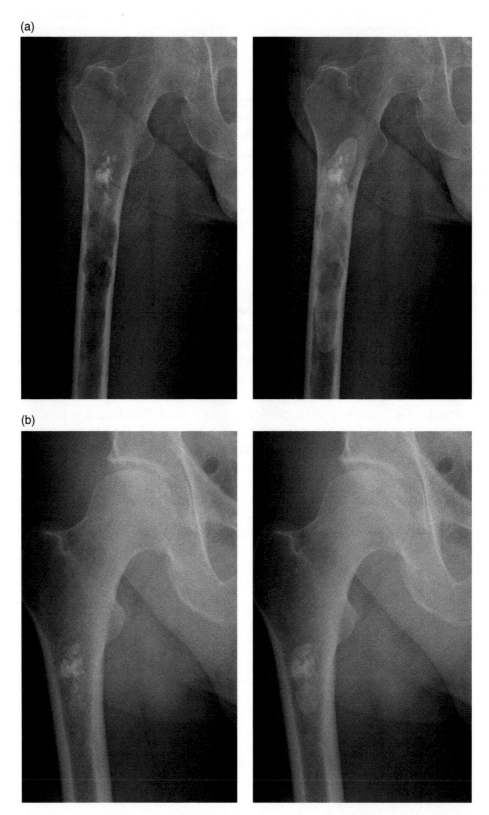

Figure 4.12 Chondrosarcoma of the proximal right femur. (a) A 68-year-old man with an insidious onset of aching in the thigh. The X-ray shows an elongated lesion with a chondroid pattern of calcification proximally and lucent appearance distally. The endosteal surface of the cortex has a scalloped appearance reflecting gradual erosion by the lobulated tumour. Although the X-ray features do not suggest a highly aggressive lesion, its large size and the fact that it is painful are important. Histology showed a low-grade chondrosarcoma. (b) X-ray of the same patient as shown in (a) but 5 years earlier. A small lesion can be seen in the medullary cavity of the proximal right femur. This has the typical 'popcorn' calcification of a chondroid lesion (orange). At the time of the X-ray, this was asymptomatic and diagnosed as an incidental enchondroma.

Ewing's sarcoma

This tumour arises from neuroectodermal 'round cells' in the marrow.

Most patients are between 5 and 15 years of age, and the tumour is almost unknown over the age of 40 years.

Clinically, the typical picture is of an unwell child with swelling at the tumour site and pain which is often severe. Pyrexia may occur.

The most common sites for Ewing's sarcoma are the femur, tibia, humerus, pelvis and ribs.

X-ray features

The bone texture is altered with a partially lytic appearance as tumour permeates through the bone (Figures 4.6a and 4.13). There is a wide zone of transition due to rapid growth. Unlike osteosarcoma and chondrosarcoma, Ewing's tumours are commonly diaphyseal or involve both the metaphysis and the diaphysis. A disproportionately large soft tissue mass is often present and sometimes visible due to bulging of the fat tissue planes or the skin contour at the same level as the bony changes.

Aggressive periosteal changes occur, and characteristically for Ewing's, an 'onion-skin' pattern can be seen. As the tumour enlarges, it lifts the periosteum in successive stages allowing a thin layer of new bone to be formed each time this happens.

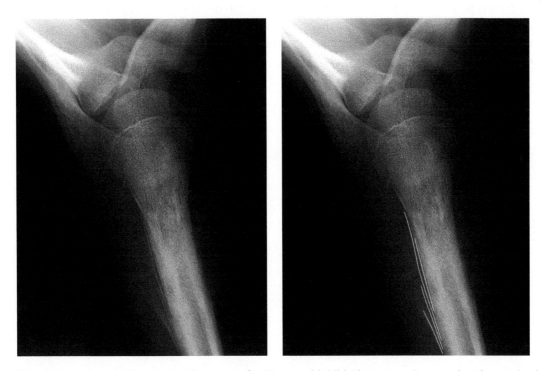

Figure 4.13 Ewing's sarcoma in the proximal humerus of a 12-year-old child. The tumour is centred at the proximal end of the diaphysis. There is sclerosis of the trabecular bone with a wide zone of transition. Periosteal new bone has an 'onion-skin' pattern due to progressive tumour enlargement (yellow).

Benign tumours

Enchondroma

An enchondroma is a benign tumour of cartilage lying within the medullary cavity of a bone.

These occur most commonly in the hands and feet.

They are often an incidental finding when the patient is X-rayed for other reasons, but presentation may also be because the patient has noticed deformity or a pathological fracture has occurred.

Enchondromas also occur outside the hands and feet in flat bones (e.g. rib), or larger long bones.

X-ray features

Enchondromas in the hands and feet are small (1–3 cm), well-defined lucent lesions centred in the medullary cavity of a metacarpal/metatarsal or phalanx (Figure 4.5b). Unlike enchondromas elsewhere, calcification within the cartilage matrix is minimal or not present. Mild bony expansion is common, along with endosteal thinning which weakens the cortex, making the bone susceptible to fracture.

Enchondromas elsewhere show similar features, but internal calcification which resembles popcorn is usually present, and cortical thinning is less of a feature (Figure 4.3).

There is a well-defined oval margin with a narrow zone of transition and no cortical destruction or periosteal reaction.

Because there is potential for malignant transformation, it can be difficult to establish whether a chondroid tumour which is not in the hands or feet is benign or malignant. Features most consistent with malignant transformation include pain, larger size (5 cm plus), a patient > 20 years of age and multiple lesions (as occur with Ollier's disease and Maffucci's syndrome).

Exostosis (Osteochondroma)

An exostosis is an outgrowth of bone with a cartilage cap. It may be pedunculated or flattened ('sessile') in shape. It is really a developmental anomaly which actively grows at the same time as the remainder of the skeleton and stops enlarging thereafter. Therefore, patients often become aware of a hard lump and present in the second decade when the normal skeletal growth spurt occurs. Sometimes, an exostosis causes mechanical symptoms for example, due to catching on a tendon or pressure on a nerve.

X-ray features

The typical site is at the metaphysis of a long bone, especially around the knee or shoulder. The cortex of the adjacent normal area of the bone is continuous with that of the osteochondroma, as is the medullary cavity (Figure 4.14).

The cartilage cap is not visible on X-ray, but it can be clearly shown on MRI. This is useful to assess malignant change which does rarely occur, presenting with pain and increased swelling. If the cap is <1 cm thick, the lesion is benign, but if it is >3 cm thick it is highly likely to be malignant. Malignant change is said to occur in 1% of solitary exostoses.

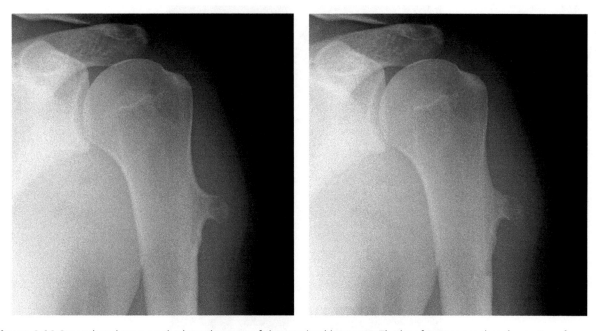

Figure 4.14 Osteochondroma on the lateral aspect of the proximal humerus. The key features are that the cortex of the exostosis is continuous with that of the surrounding normal bone (orange), as is the trabecular bone in the medullary cavity.

Osteoid osteoma

This is a small but disproportionately painful bone lesion consisting of a typically 5 to 10 mm nodule of osteoid with rich vascular and unmyelinated nerve fibre elements, surrounded by reactive bone and oedema.

A typical patient is a child or young adult complaining of unremitting pain, often causing disturbance of sleep. Seventy-five per cent of patients are between 6 and 30 years of age with a median age of 18. Common sites are the proximal femur, tibia and foot.

X-ray features

The lesion lies within the cortex, and localised smooth cortical thickening is the main feature visible on X ray (Figure 4.6b). The small, oval, lucent tumour lies within this area, but the density of the surrounding reactive bone means that it is often obscured on plain X-rays. However, it is readily demonstrated by CT (Figure 4.15). The tumour itself is often referred to as the 'nidus'. It may be partially calcified and often lies eccentrically within the sclerotic area. MRI demonstrates surrounding bone marrow oedema, which is a hallmark of this lesion.

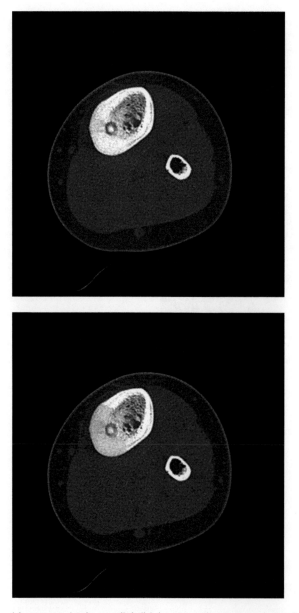

Figure 4.15 CT image of an osteoid osteoma in the medial tibial cortex. The tumour (green) is of soft tissue density with a small central calcification. The tumour itself is small in size but provokes marked thickening of the adjacent cortex (orange).

Tumour-like lesions

Fibrous cortical defect

As the name suggests, this is a lesion consisting of fibrous/fibroblastic tissue (along with osteoclasts) and is located in the cortex. It tends to be less than 3 cm in size. It is a relatively common finding on lower limb X-rays of children or adolescents as an incidental finding when the patient is X-rayed for other reasons. By early adulthood, normal bone architecture replaces the lesion, so it is virtually unseen after the age of 20 years. Because of this and the fact that it is asymptomatic, it may be regarded as a normal variant.

X-ray features

Ninety per cent occur in the lower limbs, nearly always in the tibia or femur. Fibrous cortical defects are seen in the metaphyseal region but may reach the diaphysis due to normal bone growth. A characteristic X-ray feature is that the lesion is centred in the cortex. It expands towards the medullary cavity, with a thicker inner and thinner outer layer of cortex. It is well-defined (narrow zone of transition). Larger lesions may show a 'soap bubble' appearance and also sometimes predispose to pathological fracture (Figure 4.16).

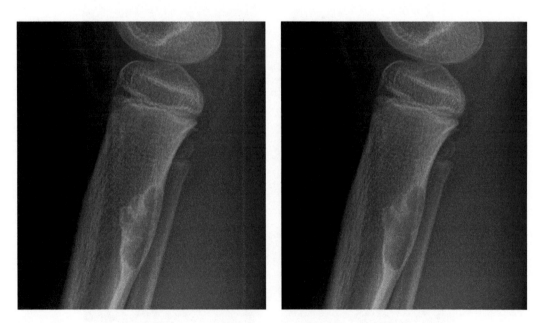

Figure 4.16 Fibrous cortical defect (red) found incidentally on an X-ray following a knee injury in a 13-year-old child. The well-defined lucent lesion characteristically expands from within the cortex, more into the medullary cavity than outwards.

Simple bone cyst

The aetiology of simple bone cysts is unknown. The lesion consists of a thin fibrous membrane lined with epithelial cells and containing fluid which is usually unilocular. The patient is typically a child between the ages of 4 and 10 years. A pathological fracture through the lesion is frequently what leads to its discovery as otherwise they are usually asymptomatic. Eighty per cent occur in the proximal femur or humerus.

X-ray features

A lucent lesion sitting centrally within the medullary cavity with a thin sclerotic margin which is often incomplete (Figure 4.17).

The site is initially metaphyseal, but they tend to migrate to the diaphysis with growth. Endosteal thinning of the cortex occurs, and there may be mild bony expansion but there is no periosteal reaction, unless this has been caused by a fracture. This may stimulate healing of the lesion.

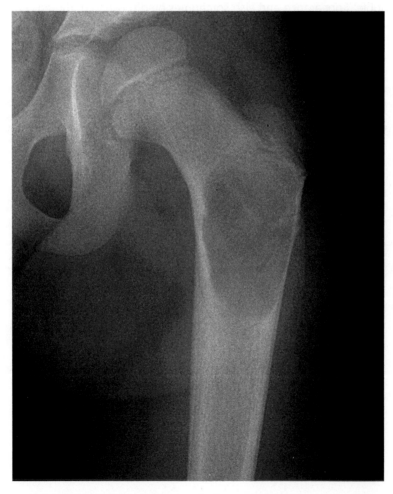

Figure 4.17 Simple bone cyst (purple) in the proximal femur of a 9-year-old child, presenting with acute pain after minor trauma. The lesion arises centrally in the medullary cavity and often presents when a pathological fracture occurs as here (red line). The radiological appearance of the lesion in this patient is almost identical to that in Figure 4.10, but a plasmacytoma does not occur in a child and a simple bone cyst is not seen in adults, emphasising how all relevant information is needed when considering the diagnosis.

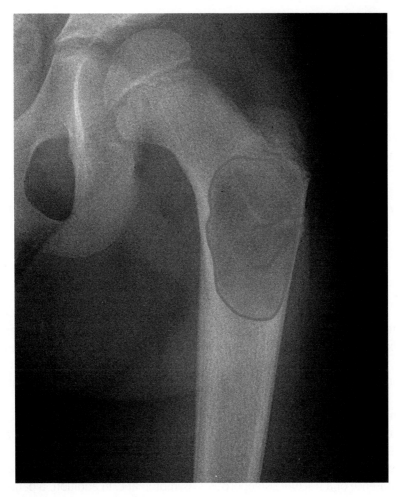

Figure 4.17 (*Continued*)

Infection

Blood-borne osteomyelitis may mimic tumour. It is seen most commonly between the ages of 5 and 15 years. Like many primary bone tumours, the infective process typically begins in the metaphyseal region and produces ill-defined bone destruction with an aggressive pattern of periosteal reaction. (This will be discussed further in Chapter 6.) Alternatively, a discrete intramedullary abscess known as a Brodie's abscess can develop. On X-ray, this shows as a localised, well-defined area of lucency with variable thickness of sclerotic margin (see Figure 6.4).

5 Metabolic bone disease

Metabolic bone disorders comprise relatively common conditions such as osteoporosis, osteomalacia secondary to nutritional deficiency of vitamin D, chronic kidney disease metabolic bone disorder (CKD-MBD) and primary hyperparathyroidism. Rarer conditions include genetic disorders such as haemochromatosis and sex-linked hypophosphataemic rickets.

These patients may present with symptoms of a low-trauma fracture but also may be identified on routine biochemical testing or following a dual-energy X-ray absorptiometry (DEXA/DXA) scan, or with characteristic X-ray findings.

Osteoporosis

Osteoporosis is a systemic skeletal disease with loss of bone mass and density leading to reduced bone strength and increased risk of fragility or insufficiency fractures. Common fracture sites are the distal radius, neck of the humerus, neck of femur, vertebral body, pubic ramus and sacral ala. It is most commonly primary in post-menopausal women but can occur in any age or sex secondary to a variety of medical problems or medications.

The disease burden and cost is high. For example, in the United Kingdom, over 2 million women have osteoporosis and 180,000 osteoporosis-related fractures occur annually with annual social and hospital care costs of £1.8 billion.

It is important to assess the risk of osteoporosis and take appropriate action to prevent fractures, but this can be difficult, as in the absence of a fracture osteoporosis is asymptomatic. In addition, a patient who has sustained one fragility fracture is at high risk of further fractures. It is therefore important to assess risk factors (e.g. older age, female, early menopause, smoking, alcohol, family history), exclude secondary causes of osteoporosis (e.g. chronic kidney disease (CKD), hyperthyroidism and corticosteroid therapy) and consider confirmation of bone mineral density (BMD) measurements with a DEXA scan. A reduction in bone density has to reach at least 30% before it can be reliably detected on X-rays.

In 2008, the guidelines for the assessment and management of fracture risk were updated by the National Osteoporosis Guideline Group (NOGG). Since this time, recommendations for further management (e.g. measuring BMD using a DEXA scan and/or starting treatment) should be based on calculating an absolute fracture risk probability within the next 10 years. The Fracture Risk Assessment Tool (FRAX) (www.shef.ac.uk/FRAX) has been validated for this purpose and uses data including independent clinical risk factors (e.g. parental history of hip fracture, alcohol intake of 4 or more units per day and rheumatoid arthritis) with or without measurement of femoral neck BMD, to calculate the 10 year probability of a major osteoporotic fracture.

Treatment for osteoporosis should always include lifestyle measures (e.g. regular weight-bearing exercise, smoking cessation and avoiding excessive alcohol intake). It is also important to ensure adequate calcium intake and vitamin D levels. Drug therapies may be indicated if the 10 year percentage probability of fracture is significant and above the NOGG treatment threshold, with bisphosphonate therapy (usually alendronate) as first-line treatment for most patients.

Musculoskeletal X-rays for Medical Students and Trainees, First Edition. Andrew K. Brown and David G. King.
© 2017 John Wiley & Sons, Ltd. Published 2017 by John Wiley & Sons, Ltd.

X-ray features

X-rays are clearly important in the diagnosis of osteoporosis-related fragility fractures. X-ray-detected sub-clinical vertebral fractures are common and indeed 50–70% of vertebral fractures do not come to clinical attention and 30% of patients over 80 have vertebral fractures. Initial X-rays in the assessment of sacral fractures or pubic rami fractures are often normal and other imaging investigations, for example isotope bone scan, MRI or CT, are more sensitive. (See also Figures 2.9, 2.32a and b, 2.35a and b, 2.36a and b, 2.38 and 2.39a and b.)

Osteomalacia

Defective bone mineralisation most commonly due to vitamin D deficiency may result in rickets in children and osteomalacia in adults. Bones may be weak and susceptible to fracture and deformity.

Vitamin D deficiency is usually caused by malabsorption, poor diet or insufficient sunlight exposure. CKD, liver disease and genetic vitamin D resistance syndromes may be additional causes.

Clinical: bone pain, fracture and proximal myopathy; possibly deformity, e.g. genu valgum or varum (knock-knees or bow-legs) in rickets.

Blood tests typically demonstrate low vitamin D, low calcium, low phosphate, high ALP and high PTH. Management involves replacing vitamin D through dietary supplementation, usually in combination with calcium.

X-ray features

X-rays may show demineralisation and loss of cortical bone, insufficiency fractures (Figure 5.1), deformity and pseudofractures called Looser's zones with transverse lucencies without bony displacement in sites such as medial proximal femur (Figure 5.2), lateral scapula and pubic rami.

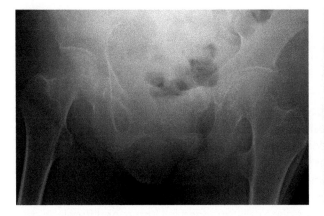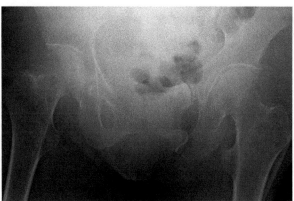

Figure 5.1 Osteomalacia with insufficiency fractures of the left superior and inferior pubic rami (orange) as well as generalised demineralisation including thinning of cortical bone.

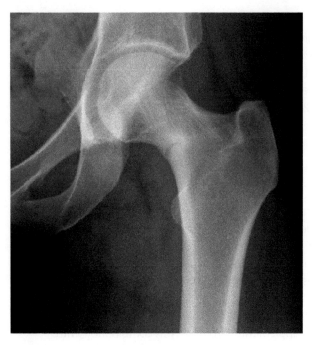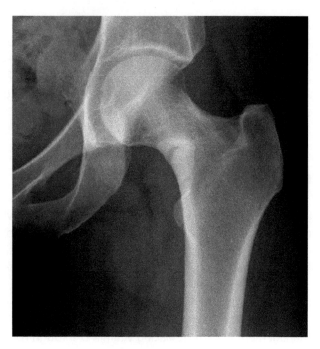

Figure 5.2 There is a diagonal cortical lucency in the medial aspect of the left femoral neck (pink) with surrounding sclerosis (yellow), consistent with a Looser's zone.

Hyperparathyroidism

This condition is caused by excess parathyroid hormone due to overproduction by the parathyroid glands, for example adenoma, hyperplasia or carcinoma (primary) or as a physiological response to low calcium levels due to, for example, low vitamin D or CKD (secondary).

Often patients are asymptomatic with raised calcium being detected as an incidental finding on a blood test. They may present with non-specific symptoms or manifestations of hypercalcaemia, for example renal stones, bone pain, myalgia, osteoporosis, nausea, vomiting, abdominal pain, constipation, polyuria and depression ('*stones, bones, abdominal groans and psychiatric moans*').

High PTH can have harmful effects on the skeleton stimulating osteoclast activity causing excess bone resorption and in extreme cases fibrous replacement and the formation of lucent 'brown tumours' in bone. Histologically brown tumours are characterised by numerous giant cells, arranged in clusters or diffusely, in a background of mononuclear oval to spindle stromal cells. Subperiosteal bone resorption may occur at various sites, particularly the phalanges. Generalised demineralisation by release of calcium from bone can further weaken bones contributing to osteoporosis and increased risk of fracture, bone pain and deformity. Treatment depends on the cause but may require surgical parathyroidectomy to remove parathyroid adenoma.

X-ray features

X-rays may demonstrate chondrocalcinosis, osteopenia, brown tumours and bone resorption. Characteristically bone resorption affects the tufts of the distal phalanges and also the subperiosteal bone on the radial aspect of the middle phalanges of the longer fingers (Figure 5.3a and 5.3b).

(a)

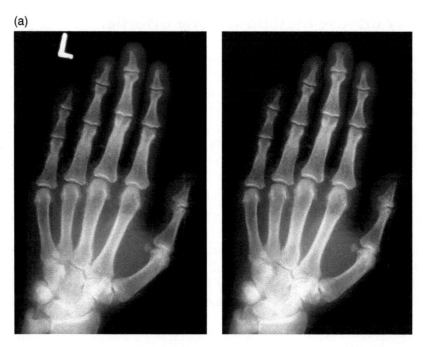

Figure 5.3 (a) Hyperparathyroidism with chondrocalcinosis of the triangular fibrocartilage in the ulna-carpal compartment of the left wrist (yellow) plus resorption of the terminal tufts of the distal phalanges (acro-osteolysis) (blue).

(b)

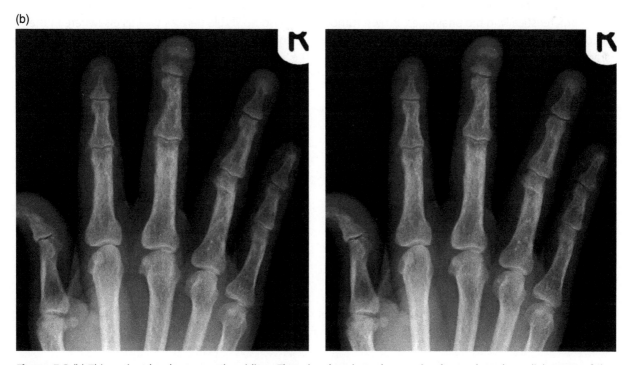

Figure 5.3 (b) This patient has hyperparathyroidism. There is subperiosteal resorption (orange) on the radial aspect of the middle phalanges of the middle and ring fingers. Also there is resorption of the distal phalanges of the index and middle fingers.

Chronic kidney disease metabolic bone disorder

CKD-MBD (also referred to as renal osteodystrophy) may become apparent in patients with CKD stages 4 or 5 after finding raised levels of phosphate and parathyroid hormone (PTH) and/or reduced levels of calcium.

Aetiology: Four mechanisms: hypocalcaemia, increased bone turnover due to secondary and tertiary hyperparathyroidism, acidosis and protein malnutrition.

Clinical: Increased fracture risk (BMD may be normal or reduced on DEXA scan); low calcium, high phosphate, high alkaline phosphatase (ALP) and high PTH.

Note: It may be a challenge to distinguish CKD-MBD from osteoporosis as both may present with low-trauma fractures and reduced BMD on DEXA scan.

Management: The two main treatment goals in CKD-MBD are as follows:

1. Achieve neutral phosphate balance through a combination of dietary restriction and use of phosphate binders.
2. Prevent secondary and ultimately tertiary hyperparathyroidism: the main driver is impaired conversion of 25-hydroxy vitamin D to the biologically active 1,25-dihydroxy vitamin D reflecting decreased activity of renal 1-alpha hydroxylase by the diseased kidney. This has led to the use of activated forms of vitamin D in CKD-MBD such as alfacalcidol and calcitriol, doses of which need to be carefully titrated against calcium levels.

Note: If using bisphosphonate drugs to treat osteoporosis be aware that they may accumulate in CKD so must be used with caution.

X-ray features

X-rays may demonstrate a variety of signs related to metabolic abnormalities and complications of CKD e.g. low vitamin D or hyperparathyroidism, making it difficult to make a definite diagnosis on the basis of the X-ray appearances alone. A wide variety of appearances may be present depending on the stage, severity and duration of CKD (Figure 5.4). Localised osteopenia may be any early sign followed by more generalised demineralisation or even insufficiency fracture or Looser's zones (Figure 5.2). Subperiosteal resorption may occur characteristically in the phalanges. Brown tumours may also be visible here as well as elsewhere in the skeleton. Bone sclerosis may occur, for example in the spine adjacent to the endplates of the vertebrae giving a characteristic 'rugger jersey' striped appearance. Signs in the soft tissues may also be visible, for example, chondrocalcinosis in the fibrocartilage of wrists or knees or more confluent soft tissue calcification (Figure 5.5).

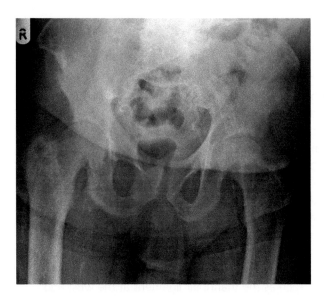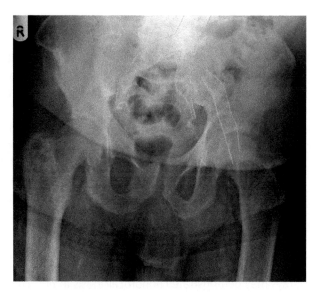

Figure 5.4 CKD-MBD. This is a patient with dialysis dependent CKD. Note the diffusely abnormal bone texture which is coarse and somewhat ill-defined in all areas (compare with normal X-ray of pelvis), in keeping with a disease process affecting all the bone suggesting a systemic metabolic bone disease. Also note the extensive calcification within the vessel of the iliac arteries within the pelvis (pink).

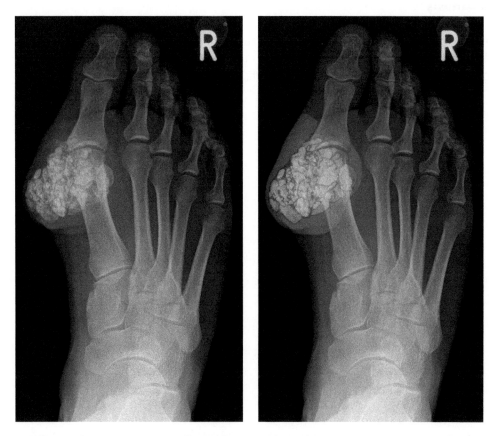

Figure 5.5 CKD-MBD. Renal tumoral calcinosis affecting the right foot, with slow progressive deposition of calcium and phosphate (yellow) and associated swelling in the subcutaneous soft tissues (green) around the first metatarsal in a patient with dialysis-dependent CKD.

Haemochromatosis

This inherited disorder of iron metabolism may result in excess iron deposition in body tissues including bones, joints, liver, pancreas and heart, which can result in damage and organ dysfunction. The diagnosis is often delayed until middle age as a result of slow progressive iron deposition and initial non-specific symptoms. Patients may present first with joint symptoms and characteristic X-ray findings leading to the diagnosis.

Musculoskeletal manifestations usually involve chronic progressive joint pain and stiffness, usually with few clinical features of inflammation. Proximal interphalangeal and metocarpophalangeal (MCP) joints of the hands (especially second and third MCPs) are typically involved, but other larger joints such as wrists, knees, hips, shoulders and feet may be affected. The pattern is usually symmetrical and can be polyarticular.

Haemachromatosis arthropathy is usually treated symptomatically with analgesics, NSAIDs and intra-articular corticosteroids and usually does not respond to removal of excess iron by venesection, particularly in cases of permanent joint damage.

X-ray features

X-rays may demonstrate chondrocalcinosis in fibrocartilage such as the triangular ligament at the wrist and menisci of the knees. Features of haemochromatosis arthropathy may resemble osteoarthritis with joint space narrowing, subchondral cysts and osteophyte formation which may be more prominent resembling a 'hook or beak-like' appearance. However the distribution of the joints involved usually differs from OA. Joint space loss may be asymmetrical. Progressive joint destruction with deformity and subluxation may occur over time.

Chondrocalcinosis

- Chondrocalcinosis is calcification of the fibrocartilage and/or hyaline cartilage
- Typical sites include knees, triangular fibrocartilage in the wrist, pubic symphysis
- Common causes include CPPD, hyperparathyroidism, haemochromatosis

---

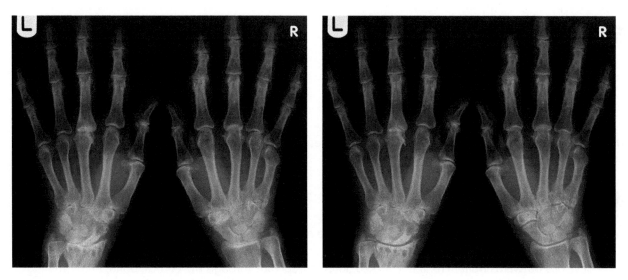

Figure 5.6 Haemochromatosis polyarthropathy of hands and wrists particularly affecting second and third fingers and carpus. There is severe joint space narrowing particularly at both third MCPJs (blue), particularly on the left, with subchondral cysts (orange) and beak-shaped osteophyte formation (yellow). Similar changes can be seen throughout the carpus and in both second and third PIPJs. Chondrocalcinosis can also be seen in the triangular fibrocartilage in the ulna-carpal compartment of the wrists (pink). Note relative sparing of DIPJs and first CMC joints commonly affected in osteoarthritis.

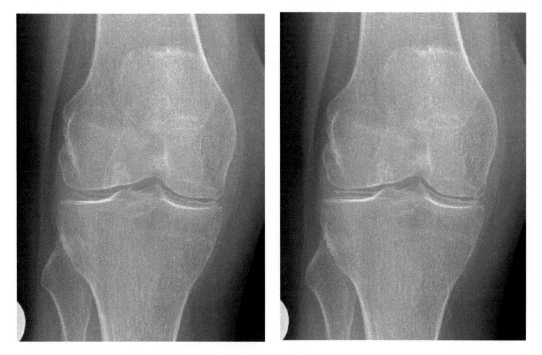

Figure 5.7 Haemochromatosis with chondrocalcinosis in the right knee.

6   Infection

This chapter covers three forms of infection which may affect musculoskeletal structures, namely osteomyelitis, septic arthritis and infective discitis.

Routes of spread

Infection may enter the bones or joints by three possible routes:

1. **Haematogenous spread**: Bacteria initially lodge in the medullary cavity, and the infective process develops outwards from here. If unchecked, infection spreads through the cortical bone, under the periosteum and into the surrounding soft tissues. It is the most common cause of osteomyelitis in children, in whom the tubular bones are usually affected. Osteomyelitis often commences in the metaphysis and may spread to involve the adjacent joint.
2. **Direct spread into bone from infection in the adjacent soft tissues**: Examples of this are seen in diabetic patients with foot ulcers and immobile patients with bedsores.
3. **Direct inoculation**: For example, from a penetrating injury, surgery or a joint injection.

Causative organisms

Gram-positive organisms account for the majority of bone and joint infections, particularly *Staphylococcus aureus*. Beta-haemolytic streptococci also contribute, especially in neonates. Anaerobes may be present in diabetic foot bone infections. *Pseudomonas* is a common organism in drug addicts. *Neisseria gonorrhoea* is also a cause of septic arthritis in young adults.

Musculoskeletal X-rays for Medical Students and Trainees, First Edition. Andrew K. Brown and David G. King.
© 2017 John Wiley & Sons, Ltd. Published 2017 by John Wiley & Sons, Ltd.

Osteomyelitis

Clinical presentation

A patient with osteomyelitis usually presents with increasing pain at the affected site. The pain may be worse with weight-bearing but unrelieved by rest. Over time, warmth, swelling and tenderness develop and the patient may feel generally unwell. Typically, the patient has a raised temperature, erythrocyte sedimentation rate (ESR), C reactive protein (CRP) and white blood cell count.

X-ray features

X-rays are usually normal for up to 3 weeks from the onset of symptoms. In the case of osteomyelitis developing from haematogenous spread, the first abnormality is often hazy reduction in bone density at the affected site. Trabecular bone is then destroyed resulting in ill-defined lytic areas in the medullary cavity, with a wide zone of transition between normal and abnormal bone. Areas of cortical destruction follow (Figure 6.1). Periosteal reaction then develops as the infective process spreads out into the adjacent soft tissues (Figure 6.2). This new periosteal bone may be incomplete and therefore have an 'aggressive' appearance if the infection is not treated. In children, the periosteum is less well bound to the cortex allowing a sub-periosteal abscess to develop more readily.

Depending on the anatomical site, swelling in the surrounding soft tissues may be visible on plain films, with loss of clarity of fat planes due to oedema and outward bulging of the skin surface. If bony infection develops as a result of spread from an adjacent soft tissue lesion, the bone changes will of course develop from the outside inwards. Periostitis and cortical destruction occur initially, followed by lytic areas in the medullary bone at a later stage (Figure 6.3).

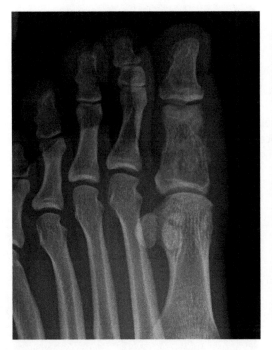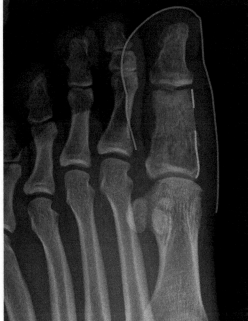

Figure 6.1 Early osteomyelitis of the proximal phalanx of the great toe. The signs are subtle: there is an area of ill-defined lucency in the medullary cavity (purple) and a breach of the adjacent cortex (adjacent intact cortex in yellow). The soft tissues of the toe are diffusely swollen (outlined in green).

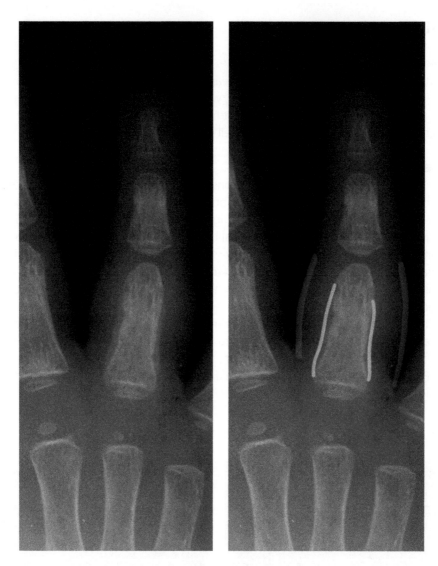

Figure 6.2 Haematogenous osteomyelitis of the proximal phalanx of a finger in a child. The infective process has spread to involve the cortex resulting in a less clearly defined appearance when compared with that of the adjacent digit and the development of surrounding periosteal new bone (yellow). The surrounding soft tissues are swollen (outlined in green).

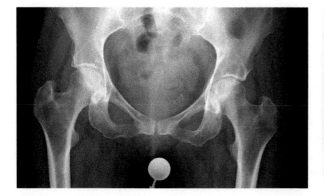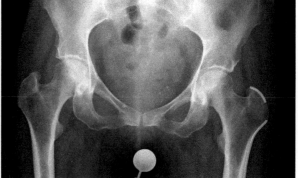

Figure 6.3 Osteomyelitis of the left greater trochanter caused by direct spread from an infected ulcer on the lateral aspect of the proximal thigh. There is focal destruction of an area of cortex (adjacent intact cortex in yellow) and of the underlying trabecular bone (orange). Compare these abnormalities with the normal right side.

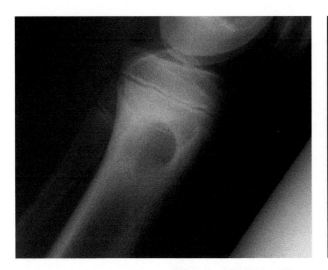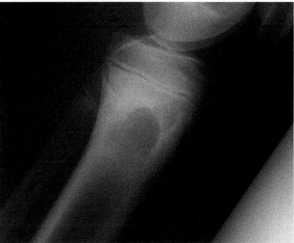

Figure 6.4 Lateral X-ray of the proximal tibia of a child showing a Brodie's abscess in the metaphysis. The margin of a Brodie's abscess typically has a well-defined, sclerotic inner demarcation but blends with the surrounding trabecular bone on its outer aspect.

Incompletely treated osteomyelitis may lead to the formation of a chronic intraosseous collection known as a Brodie's abscess. This is often found in the metaphysis of a long bone (Figure 6.4).

Other changes seen in chronic osteomyelitis include diffuse course bone architecture with thickened trabeculae and cortex. The bone may also have a generally expanded appearance due to chronic periosteal reaction (Figure 6.5a and b).

MRI has advantages over X-rays for investigating osteomyelitis. It shows infective changes in the marrow at an earlier stage. MRI also demonstrates both intraosseous and soft tissue abscesses, defining the relationship of any collections to the surrounding anatomy. This in turn allows treatment decisions on whether drainage is necessary and enables planning of the best approach (Figure 6.6).

The infective process in osteomyelitis may leave a residual fragment of avascular bone (sequestrum) within the infected area. This acts in the same way as a foreign body preventing clearing of infection. MRI or X-rays may show a sequestrum, visible as a denser bony fragment, but CT is more sensitive for demonstrating calcified abnormalities such as this and so may also sometimes be used for surgical planning.

(a)

(b)

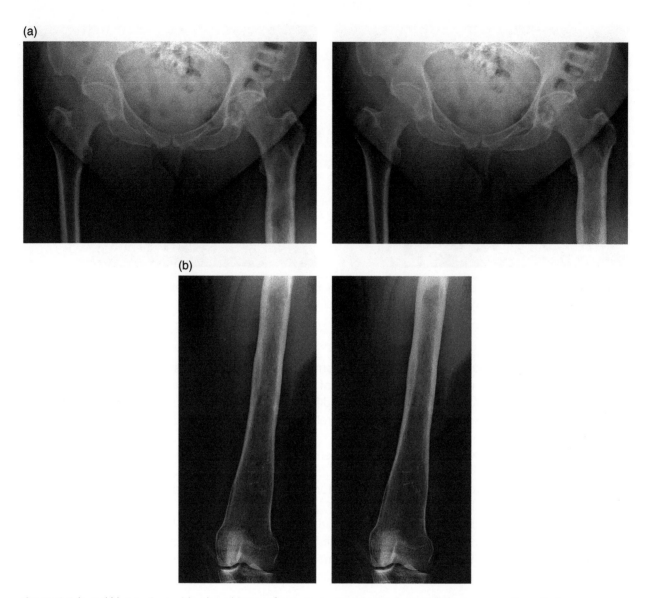

Figure 6.5 (a and b) A patient with a long history of recurrent osteomyelitis in the left femur, currently suffering an exacerbation of symptoms. Background chronic osteomyelitis changes of expansion and increased bone density are present caused by long-standing periosteal thickening (green) – compare the right and left femurs (a). There are areas of lucency (orange) in the medullary cavity due to recurrent infection. Elsewhere the trabeculae in the medullary cavity have an abnormally coarse appearance.

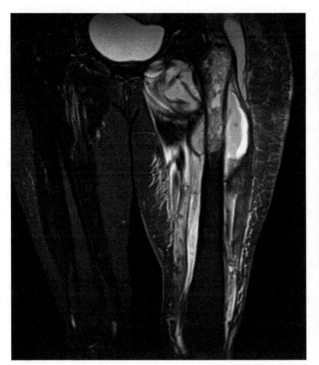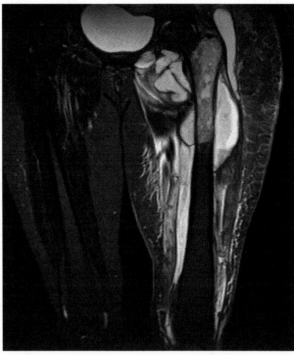

Figure 6.6 This is an MRI scan with a short TI inversion recovery (STIR) sequence which suppresses the fat signal, carried out in the same patient as Figure 6.5. High-signal areas (orange) in the proximal femoral shaft indicate active osteomyelitis. There is also extensive spread of infection into the surrounding soft tissues, producing abscesses medially and laterally (yellow).

Septic arthritis

Bacterial infection within a joint is an emergency which requires urgent diagnosis and treatment. The aim is to minimise destruction of the articular surfaces and avoid subsequent osteoarthritis. Early joint aspiration, which can be aided if required using ultrasound or X-ray screening, allows a sample of joint fluid to be obtained for microscopy, culture and sensitivity and should always be performed if the diagnosis is suspected, prior to prompt commencement of appropriate antibiotic treatment.

Clinical presentation
The clinical picture is usually of an acutely hot, swollen and tender joint. The presentation may be similar to osteomyelitis, but in addition movement is usually severely restricted due to pain. Note if the patient is immunosuppressed, the clinical presentation may be more non-specific.

X-ray features
X-rays are usually normal at the time of presentation. Also the X-ray features of septic arthritis may be indistinguishable from those of inflammatory arthritis.

The earliest X-ray change will be joint swelling if the joint affected is one where this can be visualised, such as the knee or ankle. (See the X-ray signs of joint swelling in Chapter 2.) Swelling of the adjacent soft tissues may also be visible, again depending on the site. Periarticular demineralisation occurs early on, reflecting hyperaemia due to inflammation.

High pressure from intra-articular pus may occasionally show as widening of the joint space initially (e.g. at the shoulder), but as destruction of the articular cartilage and then the articular cortex progresses the joint space rapidly becomes reduced on serial X-rays (Figure 6.7a and b). Frank bone destruction progresses to involve subchondral areas and those around the margins of the articular surface. Later, the joint may become subluxed due to bone loss and damage to the supporting soft tissue structures. These changes affect the bone on both sides of the joint equally because the destructive process starts from within the joint and works outwards. In contrast a destructive lesion arising in the bone such as a metastasis, tends to cause destruction only on one side of the joint.

(a)

(b)

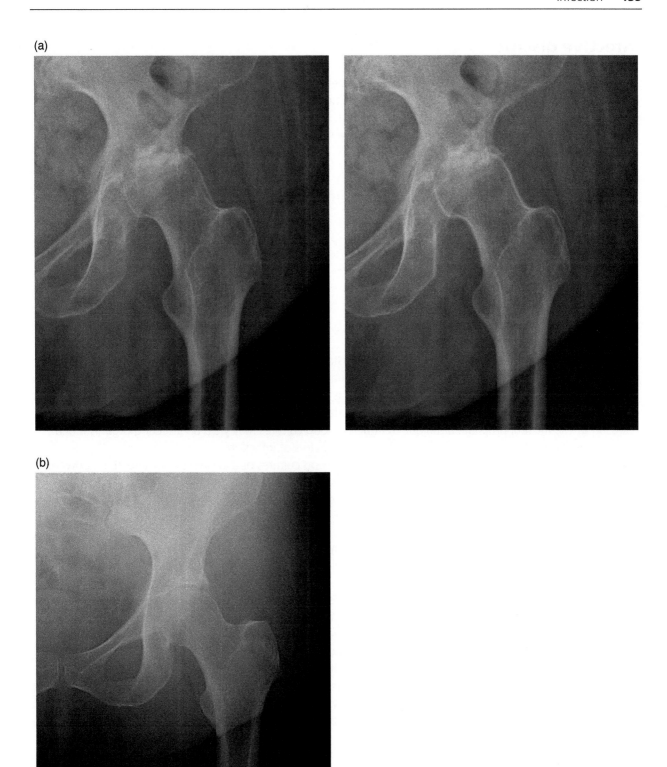

Figure 6.7 (a) X-ray of a patient presenting with severe left hip pain and rigors due to septic arthritis. There is loss of the joint space due to destruction of articular cartilage, and the articular cortex on both sides of the joint has started to be lost (incomplete adjacent cortex in yellow). This is more apparent when compared with an X-ray from 2 years earlier (b), where the cortices are intact and the femoral head has a spherical shape.

Infective discitis

The term 'infective discitis' refers to infection of the intervertebral disc and adjacent parts of the vertebral bodies. Bacteria usually reach the site via the bloodstream, initially lodging in the subcortical bone of the vertebral end plate before extending into the disc itself. Direct spread from a primary infective process in the neck, chest, abdomen or pelvis is a less common cause, as is direct inoculation from a medical procedure or an injury.

Risk factors for infective discitis:
- Recent spinal surgery
- Recent urological surgery in male patients
- Infection elsewhere
- Immunosuppression
- Diabetes
- Renal disease

Clinical presentation

Patients usually present with an insidious onset of constant (non-mechanical) back pain which is not relieved by rest or analgesia. Sometimes symptoms of back pain may be surprisingly mild and the picture is of non-specific symptoms, so having a high index of clinical suspicion is important to avoid a delay in diagnosis. ESR, CRP and white blood cell count are typically elevated. It is important to determine the causative organism to enable selection of the most appropriate antibiotic treatment. Blood cultures may yield an infecting organism and should always be obtained as culture from other potential sites of infection.

If the causative organism has not been isolated from blood cultures or a known site of infection elsewhere in the body, it is often necessary to biopsy the disc and adjacent vertebral body in order to obtain material for microscopy and culture. This is done as a radiological procedure using CT or X-ray screening guidance.

X-ray features

As with other forms of bone and joint infection, plain X-rays often show normal appearances early on in the disease. Over a few weeks, the typical changes develop. The end plates on either side of the affected disc lose clarity when compared with those at other normal levels; the disc height becomes reduced and then frank destruction of the end plates and adjacent areas of the vertebral bodies occurs. If unchecked, further bone lysis leads to loss of vertebral body height, and deformity in the form of focal kyphosis or scoliosis may develop (Figure 6.8). When discitis affects the cervical spine, prevertebral soft tissue swelling may also be seen. (The soft tissues are visible here because their anterior aspect is outlined by air in the pharynx, larynx and trachea.)

Although the X-ray features of discitis are very characteristic, they take time to become visible and it is important to diagnose and treat discitis at an early stage. Therefore, MRI is the imaging investigation of choice when the diagnosis is suspected. It will show changes when plain films are still normal and also provides precise visualisation of any associated paraspinal or extradural abscess.

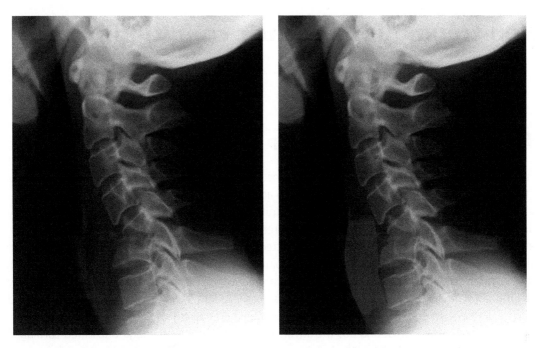

Figure 6.8 Infective discitis. The C5/6 disc 'space' has disappeared, and the vertebral body end plates on either side have been destroyed. Bone lysis due to infection is also destroying the vertebral bodies themselves (residual bone in blue) resulting in focal kyphotic deformity of the spine. There is prevertebral soft tissue swelling at the same level (orange).

7 Non-traumatic paediatric conditions

Developmental dysplasia of the hip

The term 'developmental dysplasia of the hip' (DDH) encompasses a spectrum of problems from temporary laxity of the capsular tissues in the post-natal period to an abnormally shallow acetabulum with frank posterolateral dislocation of the femoral head. The condition is multifactorial in aetiology. Family history, oligohydramnios, female sex and breech position are predisposing factors. Generally, DDH is present by the immediate postnatal period in almost all cases. If detected and treated early, there is a 95% chance of normal hip development. Otherwise, the abnormally shaped joint leads to uneven loading and subsequent early osteoarthritis. In order to avoid this, routine physical examination of all babies' hips is performed shortly after birth using the Ortolani and Barlow tests. When initial screening detects an abnormality, or there are other risk factors, the next step is an ultrasound scan. Initially, much of the anatomy of the joint is unossified and so cannot be seen on an X-ray. Ultrasound has the advantages that it is able to image unossified cartilage; it allows dynamic hip movements to be evaluated; and it also avoids ionising radiation to the pelvis.

After about the age of 4–6 months, ossification has reached the stage at which it prevents ultrasound from showing the hip structures clearly. From this age, an antero-posterior (AP) X-ray of the pelvis is used to evaluate the hips instead. X-rays are used, therefore, for later follow-up after an abnormal ultrasound examination or for late presentation of DDH.

X-ray features

The primary objective is to determine the relationship between the femoral head and the acetabulum. In DDH, the femoral head is displaced superolaterally. Looking for asymmetry between the two sides is helpful, but DDH may be bilateral in 20% of cases. When assessing the architecture of the hips, a curving line (Shenton's line) can be looked for. This normally forms a smooth arch following the medial aspect of the femoral neck and inferior aspect of the superior pubic ramus (Figure 7.1). In the case of DDH, the smooth curve is lost and (unless DDH is bilateral) Shenton's lines on the right and left sides are not symmetrical.

Next the femoral heads can be assessed. The femoral head ossification centre normally becomes visible by 6-9 months. Its appearance is often delayed in DDH so that it may smaller on the affected side.

The position of the femoral head is of primary importance. Its position can be checked by drawing two straight lines on the image (Figure 7.2a).

In DDH, the angle of the acetabular roof is abnormally steep. This is normally <30° but is increased in DDH (Figure 7.2b).

X-ray Assessment of DDH
1. Symmetry, including Shenton's lines
2. Position of femoral head – Hilgenreiner's and Perkin's lines (Figure 7.2)
3. Femoral head ossification centre
4. Acetabular angle

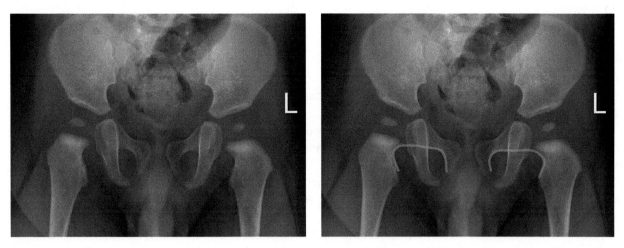

Figure 7.1 Normal pelvis X-ray at the age of 8 months. On each side, Shenton's line (green) runs along the underside of the superior pubic ramus and down the medial aspect of the femoral neck. These form two smooth symmetrical arches. The femoral head ossification centres (orange) are both present, similar in size and have a similar relationship to the acetabula.

(a)

(b)

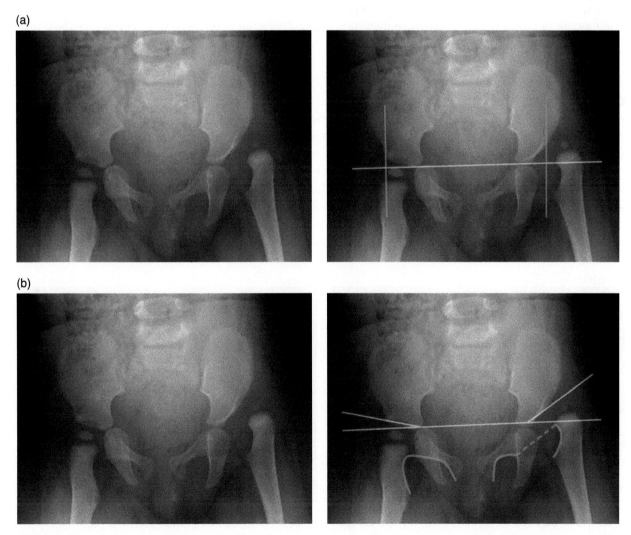

Figure 7.2 (a) An 8-month-old child with developmental dysplasia of the hip (DDH) on the left side. Note the femoral head ossification centres (orange), that on the left is smaller. The position of the femoral head at each hip is checked by drawing two lines. The first line runs horizontally through the triradiate cartilage of both acetabula (Hilgenreiner's line – white). The second line runs vertically down from the lateral aspect of the acetabulum (Perkin's line – green). Normally, the head should lie in the inferomedial quarter of the grid that these lines create, as on the right. DDH on the left causes the femoral head to lie in an abnormally superolateral position. (b) The same image as in a. The angle of the acetabular roof relative to a horizontal line through the triradiate cartilage is checked. On the left, it is abnormally steep at 40°. On the right, it is normal (under 30°). Note also the loss of the smooth curve of Shenton's line (green) on the left compared with the right.

Perthes' disease

Perthes' disease is a condition which presents with hip pain and limping in children, typically around 4–10 years old. It is four times more common in boys than girls.

The aetiology of Perthes' disease is not fully understood, but it is believed to be the result of some form of vascular insult to the femoral head. Trauma is not the cause, and the changes differ from those seen in avascular necrosis following fracture or dislocation.

Management of Perthes' disease consists of observation with intervention only when necessary. The aim is to maintain good coverage of the femoral head within the acetabulum in order to reduce the chances of secondary osteoarthritis.

Although self-limiting, the disease passes through several stages over a number of years: devascularisation of the femoral epiphysis, collapse and fragmentation, reossification and remodelling.

> **Georg Clemens Perthes** (1869–1927) was a German surgeon and a pioneer in the use of X-rays both for diagnostic purposes and cancer treatment. He initiated the use of deep X-ray therapy in 1903 and became the founder of radiological therapy in the treatment of skin cancer and carcinoma of the breast. Perthes took the first X-rays of the disease named after him in 1898.

X-ray features

At the very earliest stage, X-rays are normal, but most children do have visible changes on X-ray by the time they present. A subtle fracture line may be visible within the subchondral bone running parallel to the articular cortex of the femoral head. Later, the femoral head becomes dense and fragmented – the primary radiological signs of avascular necrosis. It may then partially collapse resulting in a flattened appearance (Figure 7.3). Healing and remodelling usually eventually leads to a return to normal appearances but when collapse of the head is severe or there is onset after 9 years of age, remodelling is more likely to be incomplete and secondary osteoarthritis may develop in adult life.

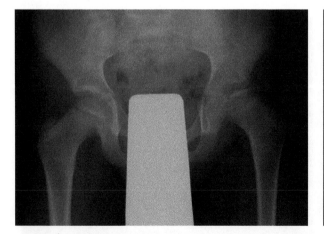 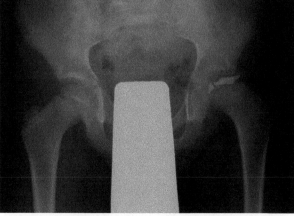

Figure 7.3 Perthes' disease of the left hip. The femoral head is dense, fragmented and shows a flattened shape (green) compared with the normal right side.

Tarsal coalition

Although it is a common cause of hindfoot pain in children and young adults, tarsal coalition often goes unrecognised initially. It is a developmental abnormality of mesenchyme in which a normal joint fails to develop. Instead, there is bridging across the joint site by bone, fibrous tissue or cartilage. The lack of movement puts abnormal focal stresses on the site of the coalition resulting in pain and stiffness.

Tarsal coalition occurs in approximately 1% of the population. There are two common sites: calcaneonavicular, which typically presents around the age of 10, and talocalcaneal, which presents in an older age group. Although the condition is congenital, its presentation a number of years after birth probably reflects progressive ossification and therefore stiffening at the coalition site.

X-ray features
Calcaneonavicular coalition is seen on the standard oblique foot projection (part of the two usual foot X-ray views taken) as an extension from the anterior calcaneum to the adjacent aspect of the navicular. There may be continuous bone bridging the space with an ossified coalition. If there is a soft tissue coalition (either fibrous or cartilaginous), the space is narrowed and the adjacent bony margins show increased sclerosis or irregularity of the cortex (Figure 7.4). Talocalcaneo coalition occurs at the joint between the sustentaculum tali, towards the medial side of the calcaneus, and the talus above. This joint is best seen on a lateral X-ray of the ankle. In the normal situation, the two bones are separated and these surfaces are smooth and corticated. If there is a bony coalition, the joint is filled in by continuous ossification. The lateral ankle view demonstrates this as the 'C-sign' (Figure 7.5a and b). When the X-ray findings are not clear-cut, a CT or an MRI can provide further detail and either confirm or exclude the diagnosis of coalition (Figure 7.6).

(a)

(b)

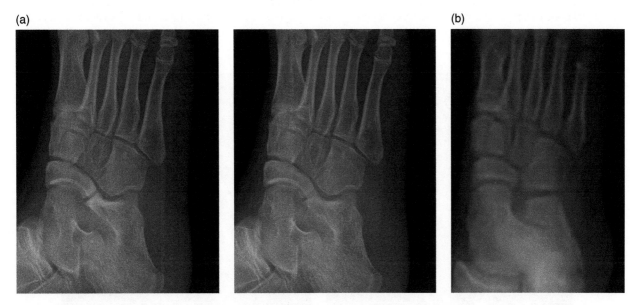

Figure 7.4 Calcaneo navicular coalition in an 11-year-old presenting with foot pain. (a) There is abnormally prominent bone extending between the anterior calcaneum and the navicular (blue). The bone at this site is sclerotic due to increased stresses caused by restriction of the normal flexibility of the foot. (b) The X-ray appearances of a normal foot in a child of the same age for comparison.

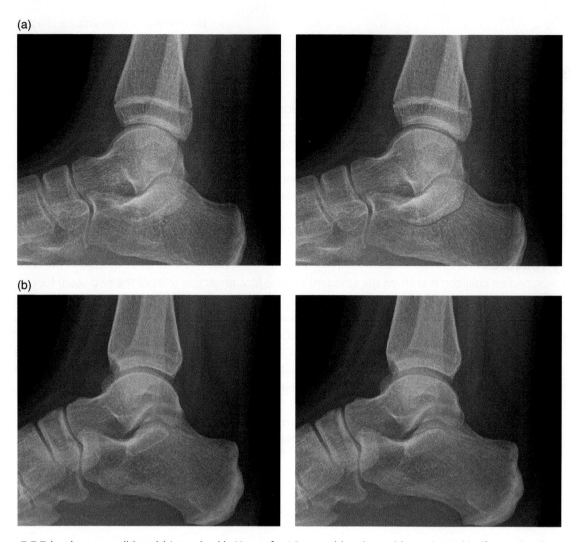

Figure 7.5 Talocalcaneo coalition: (a) Lateral ankle X-ray of a 16-year-old patient with persistent hindfoot pain. There is no visible gap at the posterior aspect of the joint between the sustentaculum and the talus, resulting in a continuous C-shape of cortical bone (blue). (b) Normal subtalar joint for comparison. Separate cortices of the talus and the sustentaclum are shown in orange. A space is clearly visible between the articular surfaces of the sustentaculum below and the talus above at the posterior aspect of the joint.

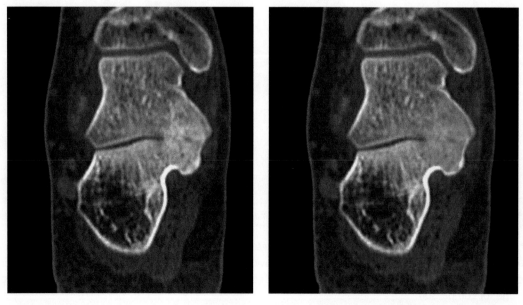

Figure 7.6 Coronal CT slice through the hindfoot showing abnormal ossification (blue) between the sustentaculum tali and the talus, in place of the normal joint.

Osteochondritis dissecans

Osteochondritis dissecans is a condition in which a focal area of damage develops in the articular cartilage and underlying epiphysis of a growing bone. Common sites are the lateral side of the medial femoral condyle at the knee and the capitellum at the elbow.

It is seen in both male and female patients, mainly between the ages of 10 and 20 years. The aetiology is not fully understood, but there may be an element of vascular insufficiency and also repetitive focal trauma may play a role as the condition has an association with sports, for example the elbow lesion in gymnastics.

X-ray features
A focal area of lucency is seen in the subchondral bone of the epiphysis (Figure 7.7). Irregular ossification and fragmentation may develop, and in some cases the affected osteochondral fragment becomes unstable and separates to become a lose body within the joint.

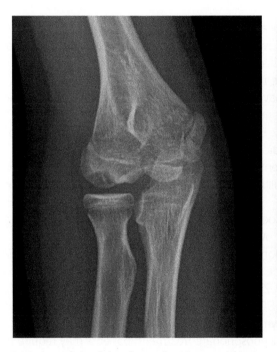
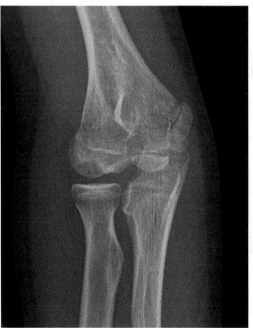

Figure 7.7 AP view of the right elbow of a 10-year-old keen gymnast, with chronic aching laterally. There is an approximately 1 cm diameter area of focal lucency in the capitellum (orange). Combined with this history the features are typical of osteochondritis dissecans.

8   Other bone pathology

In this chapter, we have included three other bone disorders which are more difficult to specifically classify but are sufficiently common and relevant to routine clinical practice:

- Paget's disease of bone (PDB)
- Hypertrophic Osteopathy (HOA)
- Avascular necrosis (AVN) (also called osteonecrosis)

Paget's disease of bone

PDB is a disorder of unknown cause characterised by localised sites of disorganised bone metabolism with excess bone reabsorption and new bone formation followed by bone remodelling. Bones may enlarge and reduce in strength, resulting in pain, fracture and arthritis.

Most commonly affected bones are the pelvis, femur, tibia, skull and lumbar spine.

Up to 3% of the UK population over 55 years may have PDB, but there are large geographical variations. Males are most commonly affected. Genetic factors (genes identified in 25%) and viral infections (e.g. paramyxoviruses) have been implicated in the aetiology. PDB is usually diagnosed from a combination of an isolated elevation in alkaline phosphatase (ALP) and typical radiological features.

Clinical presentation: Frequently asymptomatic incidental finding, bone pain, osteoarthritis (OA), pathological fracture, bone deformity, hearing loss (skull base PDB), cord compression (vertebral PDB) and rarely osteosarcoma.

Investigations: blood tests: raised ALP due to bone isoenzyme (may be an isolated chance test finding); imaging: x-ray diagnostic, isotope bone scan useful for overall distribution and baseline assessment.

Management: The main indication for treatment is bone pain. The newer amino-bisphosphonate drugs such as alendronate, risedronate and zoledronate (ZA) are the treatments of choice and work by suppression of metabolic activity through decreased osteoclast activity. ZA is probably the most commonly used and effective, with a single intravenous dose resulting in remission in 90%, which can continue for several years or even long term. Re-treatment is now usually based on return of symptoms rather than serial checking of ALP.

Whereas bone pain due to PDB is an indication for bisphosphonate treatment, patients may require further radiological assessment to confirm that the pain is caused by active PDB as opposed to a complication such as osteoarthritis.

X-ray features

During the active phase, there is lucency of the affected area with well-defined margins which in the skull gives rise to the term 'geographic skull'. In a long bone, the margin has an edge which may resemble the shape of a flame. In the established phase, the characteristic X-ray features are coarse trabeculation, cortical thickening, bone expansion and sclerosis (Figure 8.1). Softening of the bone may lead to deformity in the weight-bearing areas of the skeleton (Figure 8.2).

Musculoskeletal X-rays for Medical Students and Trainees, First Edition. Andrew K. Brown and David G. King.
© 2017 John Wiley & Sons, Ltd. Published 2017 by John Wiley & Sons, Ltd.

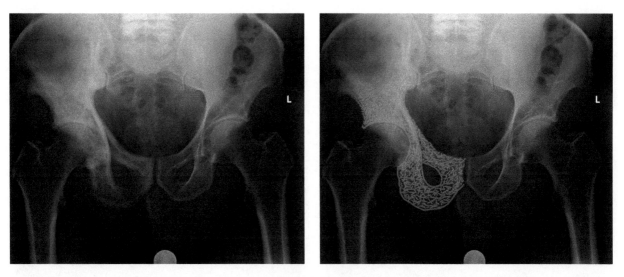

Figure 8.1 An area of PDB (blue) affecting predominantly the ischium and pubic bone in the right hemipelvis characterised by coarse trabeculation, cortical thickening, bone expansion and sclerosis. Compare these features with the normal left side.

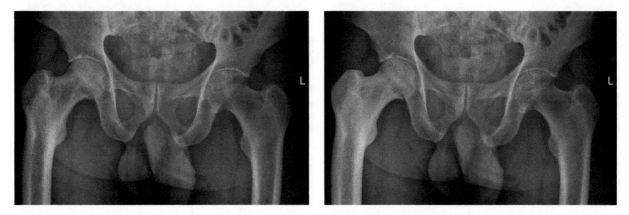

Figure 8.2 PDB affecting the right femur with cortical thickening, bone expansion and early bowing deformity (yellow). The changes are more obvious when compared to the normal appearances of the left femur.

(a)

(b)

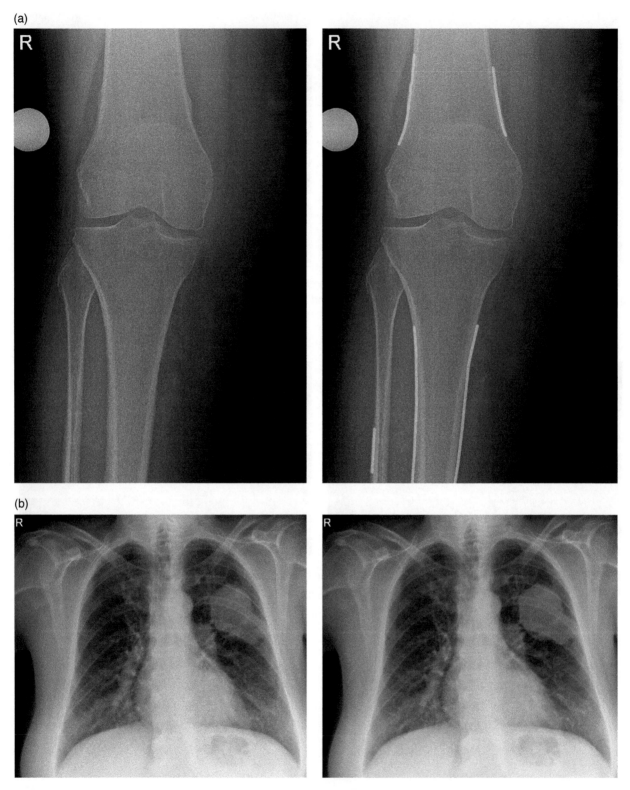

Figure 8.3 HPOA (a) There are subtle periosteal reactions shown as irregular thickening of the outer cortex (yellow) involving the distal femur, proximal tibia and fibula, which given the chest X-ray findings are typical of HPOA. (b) There is a well-circumscribed lobulated opacity in the upper zone of the left lung (orange) highly suggestive of a lung cancer.

Hypertrophic Osteoarthropathy (HOA)

This uncommon condition can occur as a primary entity of unknown cause (approximately 5%) or more usually secondary to other medical conditions particularly lung disease, including 5% of patients with lung cancer, particularly those with non–small-cell cancer. As this is the most common association, it is often also called hypertrophic pulmonary osteoarthropathy (HPOA). Other causes may include other pulmonary conditions such as mesothelioma or lung abscess, cyanotic congenital heart disease and inflammatory bowel disease.

It is characterised by periostitis which can affect small joints of the hands and long bones particularly around the ankles and wrists. Patients have pain at these sites. It is often associated with clubbing of the fingers and toes.

X-ray features
X-ray typically show a smooth incomplete periosteal reaction adjacent to joints with new bone formation involving particularly the diaphysis and metaphysis of the long bones, without any abnormality in the adjacent bone. Appearances are often visible on each side of the bone. There may be some soft tissue swelling. As the condition progresses, periosteal changes may extend a little further distally and become multi-layered with an 'onion-skin' appearance (Figure 8.3).

Avascular necrosis

This condition is characterised by loss of blood supply and subsequent death of bone cells followed by necrosis, destruction and collapse.

Any bone can be affected, but particularly the femoral head, talus, scaphoid and shafts of long bones. Single or multiple sites may be involved.

The cause is often unknown, but a number of risk factors have been associated with AVN which include trauma, chemo- or radiotherapy, alcohol excess, bone marrow pathology, decompression sickness from diving and drug treatments including corticosteroid and bisphosphonates (which is particularly associated with AVN of the jaw). Interestingly, the condition can often be asymptomatic or present with pain in the affected site of variable intensity.

X-ray features
X-rays are typically normal in the early stages of this condition, and MRI and isotope bone scan are more sensitive initial imaging investigations. Mild osteopenia may be the first radiographic sign. Bone resorption occurs and the affected bone may appear more radio-opaque with subchondral sclerosis, with subsequent subchondral bony collapse which may lead to the appearance of a 'crescent sign' with subchondral lucency in the femoral head which may lose its usual spherical shape with cartilage destruction leading to secondary degenerative arthropathy. The characteristic features of established AVN are fragmentation and increased density of the affected area of bone.

(a)

(b)

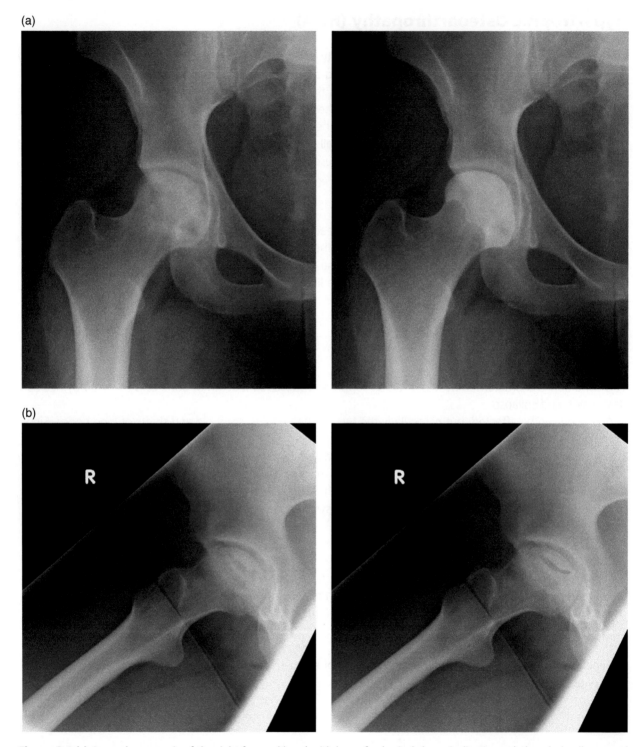

Figure 8.4 (a) Avascular necrosis of the right femoral head with loss of spherical shape indicating subchondral collapse and areas of increased density bilaterally (yellow). Note that the joint space is preserved, and there is no abnormality on the acetabular side of the joint as the pathological process is within the femoral head. (b) Lateral right hip X-ray demonstrating the 'crescent sign' indicating a fracture of the subchondral bone of the femoral head (orange).

9 Joint replacement

Arthropathy, especially osteoarthritis of the hip and knee, is highly prevalent among older adults. Joint replacement or arthroplasty is a very successful treatment once more conservative measures are no longer sufficient to control symptoms. As a result, it is now common to encounter joint replacements in everyday practice, and therefore, it is useful to be aware of the normal and abnormal features of arthroplasties on X-ray and also the limitations of plain films for evaluating complications. Numerous designs of implant exist for many different joints. The joint may be completely or partially replaced, and the components might be cemented or uncemented. However, in general, arthroplasties all share the same potential complications: hardware failure, aseptic loosening, infection, malalignment, instability and periprosthetic fracture.

Hardware failure and aseptic loosening

Rarely, the metal of a prosthesis may fracture if subjected to sufficient stress. This can be appreciated on X-rays, as a change in the normal shape and continuity of the component, most commonly the neck or stem of a hip replacement. However, it is much more common for joint replacements to fail as a result of gradual wear at the joint surfaces. Many types of joint replacement use polyethylene on one side of the articulation in order to reduce friction. But friction can never be completely abolished, so over time this leads to the shedding of metal and polyethylene micro-particles from the joint surfaces. In particular, polyethylene very slowly wears down and the resulting gradual loss of thickness may be visible on sequential X-rays. Polyethylene has an X-ray density similar to soft tissue, and it might be thought of as similar to the hyaline cartilage occupying the 'joint space'.

As it wears the 'joint space' narrows, and this can be assessed by comparing X-rays taken shortly after the joint was implanted with up-to-date images (Figure 9.1a and b). Assessing polyethylene wear on plain films has limitations as the measurements vary with the exact position of the patient when the X-ray is taken and the angle of the X-ray beam.

However, it is the generation of micro-particles which is a greater problem because this is the main cause of aseptic loosening: Micro-particle debris gradually gains access into the bone, either directly against the prosthesis or between the bone and the cement, where it causes histiocytic osteolysis to occur. This process gradually erodes the layer of bone to which the prosthesis is bonded and so it becomes loose.

Loosening becomes visible on X-ray as progressive lucency around a joint replacement, either generally or in focal areas (Figure 9.2a and b and Figure 9.3a and b). As osteolysis becomes more severe around a component, its position may alter. For example, the angulation of a component may alter (Figure 9.4) or the femoral component of a hip replacement may subside down into the femur. (*Note*: one exception is that the femoral component of an *uncemented* total hip replacement (THR) may subside by up to 1 cm as a normal finding.) Fractures of the cement surrounding a component are a further sign of loosening.

These changes are usually subtle and for that reason it is essential to compare the appearances on current X-rays with those on films taken soon after the surgery was performed. It is normal to see a thin line of lucency

Musculoskeletal X-rays for Medical Students and Trainees, First Edition. Andrew K. Brown and David G. King.
© 2017 John Wiley & Sons, Ltd. Published 2017 by John Wiley & Sons, Ltd.

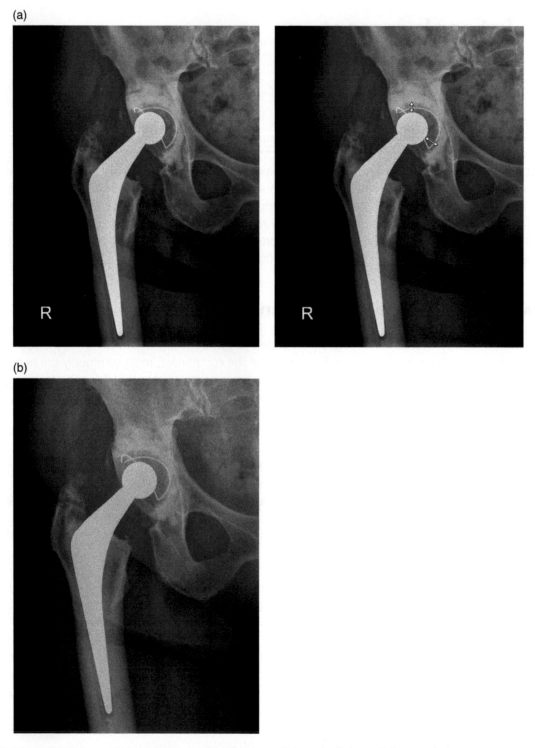

Figure 9.1 (a and b) Right total hip replacement showing wear of the polyethylene of the acetabular component: In (a) the 'space' between the metal head of the femoral component and the acetabular cement is occupied by the polyethylene cup. This shows subtle reduction in thickness superiorly compared to other areas (white arrows). There is also lucency between the cement and the bone of the acetabulum indicating loosening (blue). Both of these features have developed since an earlier normal film (b).

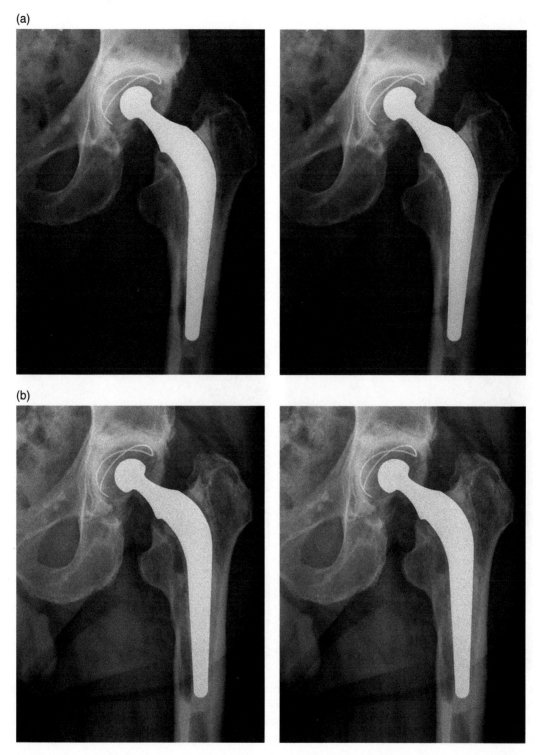

Figure 9.2 (a and b) Loosening of a femoral component: (a) The first film shows the appearances 11 years after surgery. There is an abnormally wide (i.e. >2 mm) lucent line at the junction of the cement and surrounding bone in some areas around the stem (orange). (b) An X-ray 2 years later shows that the width of the lucency has increased, indicating progressive loosening. The stem has also displaced medially away from the cement a little (green). This change in position of a component is a further sign of loosening.

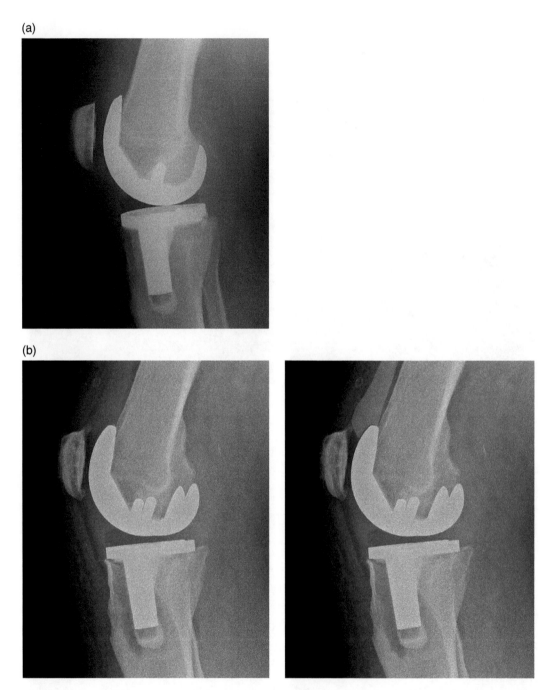

Figure 9.3 (a and b) Loosening of the tibial component of a total knee replacement. (a) The normal immediate post-operative film. The surgical staples are just visible in the anterior skin layer. (b) An X-ray 10 years later shows prominent lucency in the bone anterior to the tibial component due to osteolysis (orange). There is also swelling of the suprapatellar pouch (yellow) which would be expected immediately after surgery but should not be present at a later stage.

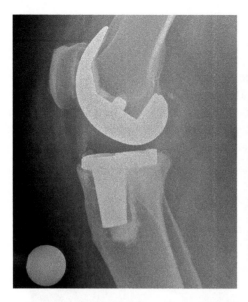
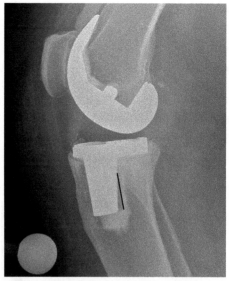

Figure 9.4 Loose tibial component showing change in position. The original position of this component is revealed by its impression in the posterior cement (black line). This was confirmed on the original post-operative films (not shown). There is now a backward tilt of the metalwork relative to the starting position indicating that it is loose. There is also swelling of the joint shown as thickening of the suprapatella pouch (yellow), a non-specific sign of a problem in the knee.

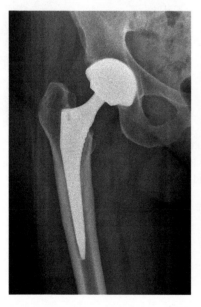
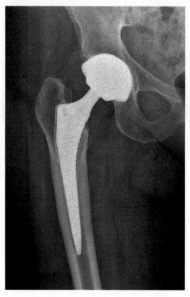

Figure 9.5 Normal appearances of an uncemented total hip replacement. In some areas, a thin lucent line (green) can be seen between the metal and the surrounding bone. This is normal if it measures less than 2 mm in width. Also the redistribution of forces in the bone has resulted in cortical thickening around the stem (blue), which is also a normal appearance.

between the cement and the surrounding bone (or between the prosthesis and the bone if it is uncemented). This lucent line should not be more than 2 mm wide in the normal situation (Figure 9.5).

Introducing a joint replacement affects the loading of the surrounding bone which responds, according to Wolff's law, with resorption in areas of reduced load and thickening where stresses are increased. For example, this is seen after an uncemented hip replacement when there is often gradual loss of bone density at the calcar (the dense area of bone present in the posteromedial femur, superior to the lesser trochanter) and an increase in thickness of the cortex around the stem as the bone responds to the redistribution of forces (Figure 9.5). These normal changes should not be mistaken for signs of loosening.

Infection

An infecting organism usually gains access at the time of operation, and therefore infection tends to manifest itself clinically within the first weeks to months after surgery. It is important to realise that plain X-rays alone are neither sensitive nor specific as a test for infection. They may either be normal or show similar features to those of aseptic loosening (Figure 9.6). Therefore, the overall assessment will include clinical evaluation, inflammatory blood markers, microbiology cultures and possible further imaging such as white cell–labelled nuclear medicine scan. Joint aspiration can be performed, aided by X-ray screening or ultrasound guidance if necessary.

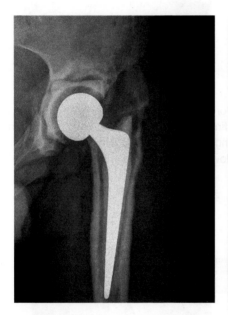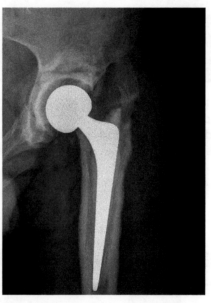

Figure 9.6 Infected total hip replacement. There is prominent lucency at the bone/cement interface of both the femoral and acetabular components (green). The femoral component is also displaced distally into the medullary cavity. These features could also be due to aseptic loosening but ultrasound-guided aspiration identified infected joint fluid.

Malalignment and instability

The positioning of individual components is an important factor in ensuring a good long-term result in joint replacement surgery, but specific details vary from prosthesis to prosthesis making this too large a subject for this book. As well as surgical technique, the final position of the joint will also be governed by soft tissue and bony factors in the individual patient.

Subluxation and dislocation is a problem which may occur with joint replacements at any site, and therefore the alignment between the two sides of the joint should be checked. The two articular surfaces of the joint prosthesis should be congruent and the centre of the articular surface on one side of the joint should line up with the centre of the component on the opposite side. This should be checked on two views at 90° to one another if dislocation is suspected and is not shown on a single view (Figure 9.7).

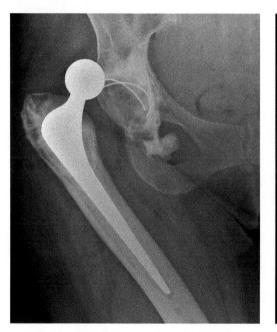 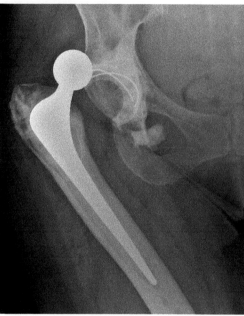

Figure 9.7 A patient with acute hip pain due to dislocation of a THR following a fall. The femoral head has displaced superolaterally and is no longer sitting in the cup (yellow), the position of which can be inferred from the marker wires incorporated into the polyethylene.

Periprosthetic fracture

This is a complication which might occur at the time of initial surgery or any time afterwards. A fracture occurring at surgery can occasionally go undetected by the surgeon and so may only come to light on post-operative check X-rays. Later periprosthetic fractures are usually easily seen (Figure 9.8) but occasionally remain undisplaced and difficult to detect, for example in the pelvis adjacent to an acetabular component in an osteoporotic patient. CT may be useful to check for a fracture in this situation.

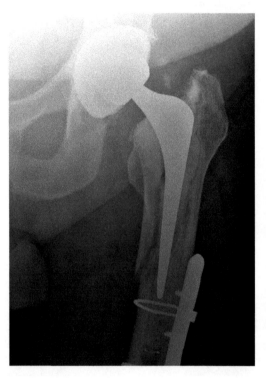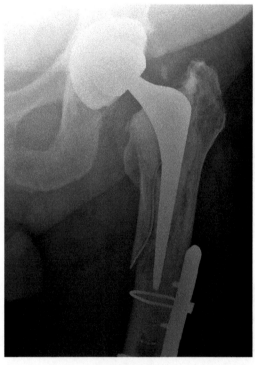

Figure 9.8 Periprosthetic fracture of the femur. There is a fracture of the proximal femoral shaft, visible as a linear lucency extending from the medial cortex proximally (orange). The patient has also undergone plating of a more distal femoral shaft fracture in the past.

PART 3

This section is an opportunity to test yourself and see further examples of X-ray findings discussed in the previous chapters. We suggest that you work through each of the cases and firstly describe each abnormality using the conventions outlined in the book before answering each question in turn. The patients' names and the dates have been removed from these images but in the real life setting these should always be checked and included when presenting images. The answers are provided later, together with annotated X-ray images.

Self-assessment questions

Case 1

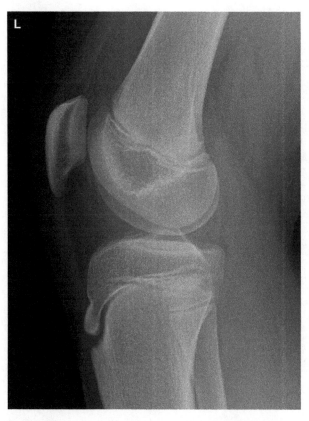

Mr A.B., aged 14 years. Posterior knee pain following an acute injury. Lateral view. The AP view was normal. No bony tenderness on examination.

Q1 Is there any bony injury?

Q2 Does the X-ray show joint swelling?

Case 2

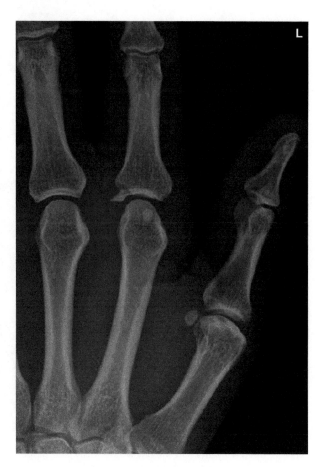

Mr C.D., aged 37 years. On the day of the X-ray, he suffered an acute injury of the left index finger from a severe valgus force. This is a magnified area from an X-ray of the left hand.

Q1 Describe the injury as shown on this view.

Q2 What action would you take if you were the emergency department doctor seeing this patient?

Musculoskeletal X-rays for Medical Students and Trainees, First Edition. Andrew K. Brown and David G. King.
© 2017 John Wiley & Sons, Ltd. Published 2017 by John Wiley & Sons, Ltd.

Case 3 (a and b)

(a)

(b)

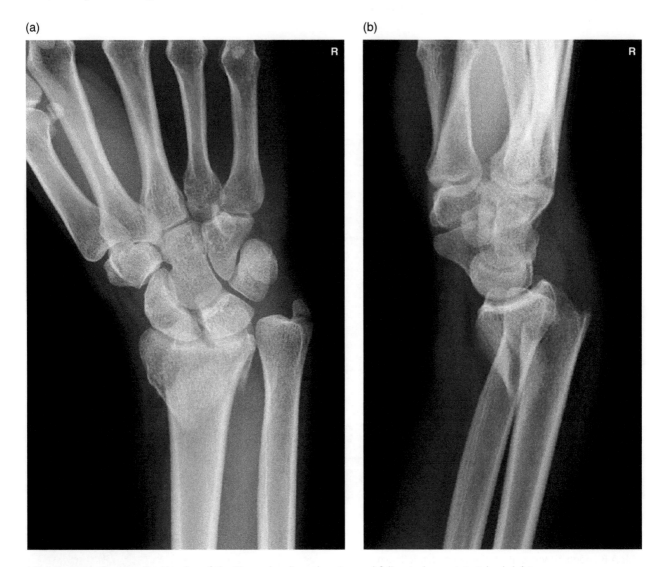

Ms E.F., aged 45 years. On the day of the X-ray, she slipped on ice and fell onto her outstretched right arm.

Q1 Describe the site(s) and orientation of the fractures.

Q2 Describe the displacement.

Case 4

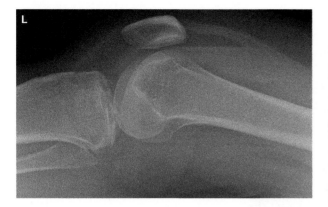

Mrs S.T., aged 49 years. Fall downstairs. Painful swollen knee. Unable to weight-bear. Horizontal-beam lateral X-ray of the left knee.

Q1 What signs are visible on this horizontal-beam lateral view?

Q2 What else do you need to complete the X-ray examination?

Case 5

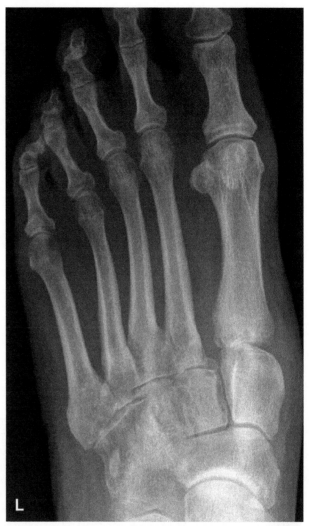

Mr G.H., aged 64 years. Three weeks earlier crashed while driving his car, injuring his left foot in the pedals. This is the dorsoplantar (straight) view of the foot.

Q1 Describe the site and displacement of any abnormality you can identify.

Q2 What other view would be helpful?

Case 6

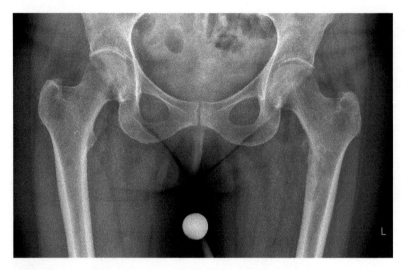

Ms I.J., aged 71 years. Insidious onset of proximal left thigh pain. Previous history of lung cancer 2 years ago.
Q1 Identify and describe the abnormality.
Q2 What is the most likely cause?
Q3 What other imaging tests might be appropriate and why?

Case 7

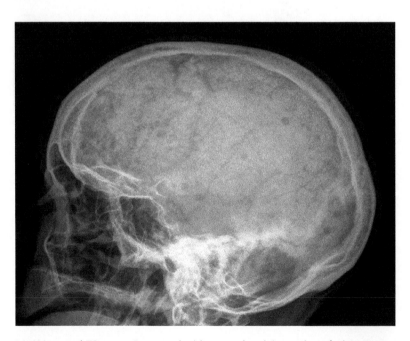

Mr K.L., aged 72 years. Presented with general malaise and confusion. Tests revealed a raised level of paraprotein in the blood and Bence Jones protein in the urine.
Q1 What is this view and why would the X-ray be taken?
Q2 Identify and describe the abnormality.
Q3 Would a radioisotope bone scan be helpful?

Case 8

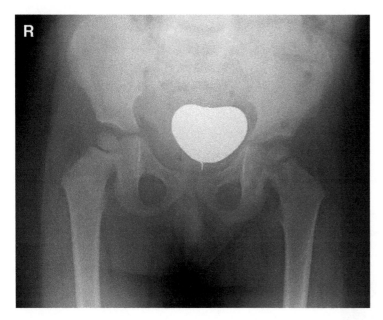

Master Q.R., aged 2 years. Worsening fever, limp and severe left hip pain over past 3 weeks.

Q1 What are the most important diagnoses to consider from the clinical presentation?

Q2 Identify and describe any abnormality on the X-ray.

Q3 What other imaging tests may be useful for diagnosis and to guide management?

Case 9

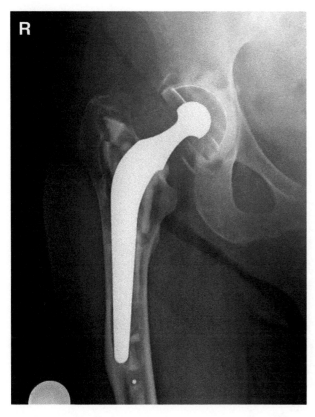

Mr M.N., aged 79 years. Right total hip replacement (THR) 14 years earlier. Increasingly painful over the past 2 years.

Q1 Describe the signs on this X-ray.

Q2 What do the signs indicate?

Case 10

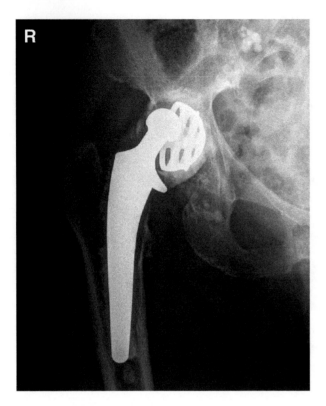

Mr O.P., aged 83 years. Presented with acute severe hip pain after suddenly twisting.

Q1 Describe the X-ray appearances.
Q2 What is the likely cause of his presentation?
Q3 What could you do to confirm your diagnosis?

Case 11

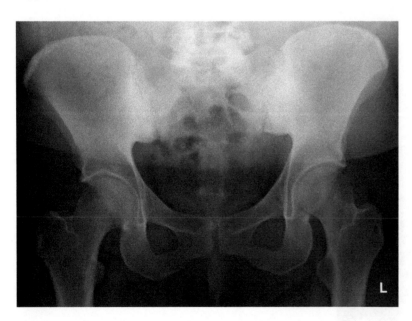

Mr Q.R., aged 35 years. Persistent lower back and buttock pain with morning stiffness.

Q1 Describe the X-ray appearances.
Q2 What is the likely diagnosis?
Q3 What additional imaging test would be useful to look for active inflammation?

Case 12

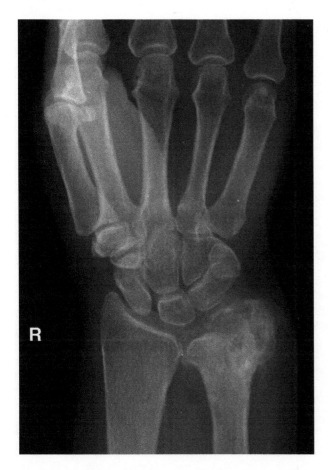

Mrs S.T., aged 74 years. Recurrent episodes of warm red swelling of the right wrist.

Q1 Describe the X-ray appearances.

Q2 What is the likely diagnosis?

Q3 How would you confirm the diagnosis?

Case 13

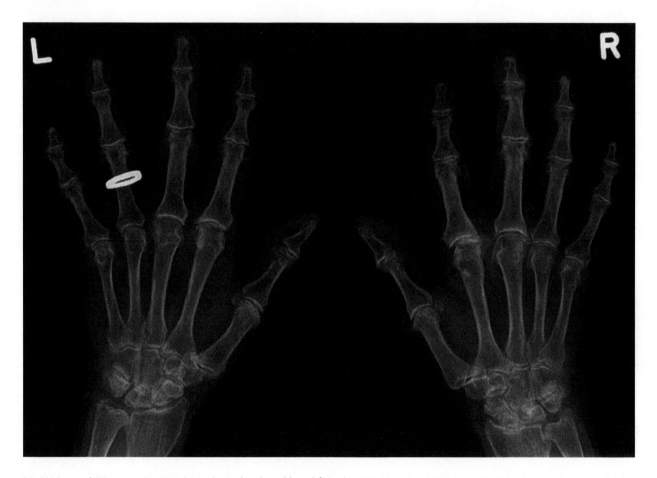

Mr U.V., aged 52 years. Progressive pain and reduced hand function.

Q1 Describe the X-ray appearances.

Q2 What is the likely diagnosis?

Q3 How would you confirm the diagnosis?

Case 14 (a and b)

(a)

(b)

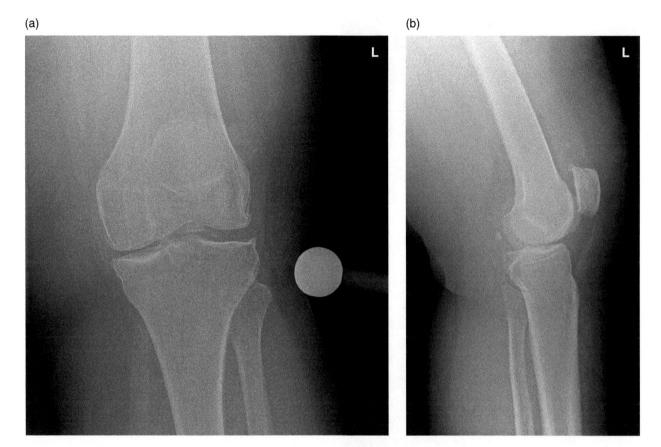

Mrs X.Y., aged 71 years. Persistent left knee pain and occasional locking.

Q1 Describe the X-ray appearances.

Q2 What is the likely diagnosis?

Case 15

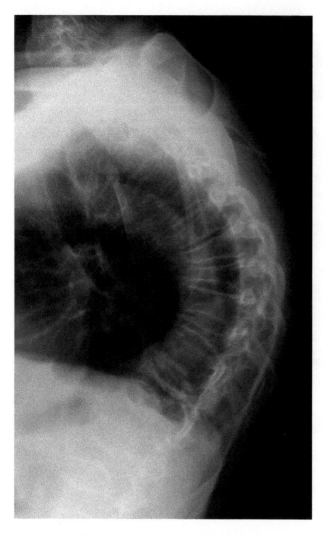

Mrs Z.A., aged 82 years. Recurrent episodes of acute
thoracic back pain and change in posture.
Q1 Describe the X-ray appearances.
Q2 What is the likely diagnosis?
Q3 What other tests may help to confirm the diagnosis?

Case 16

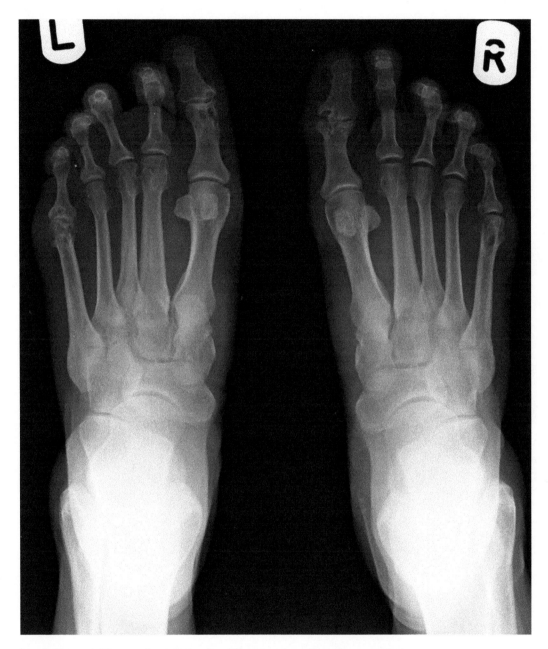

Mrs B.C., aged 46 years. Persistent pain, stiffness and swelling of symmetrical metatarsophalangeal (MTP) joints.

Q1 Describe the X-ray appearances.

Q2 What is the likely diagnosis?

Q3 What other imaging investigations may be most helpful to look for active joint inflammation?

Case 17

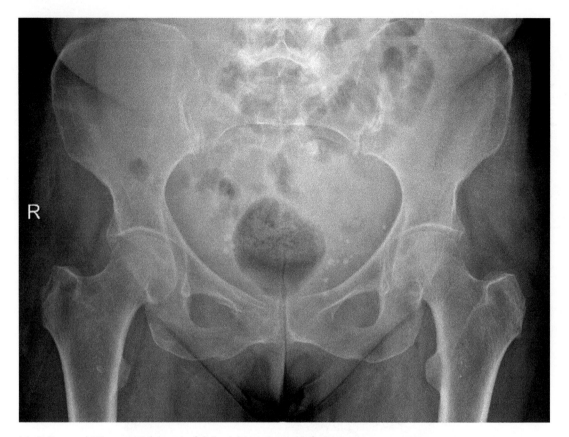

Mr D.E., aged 77 years. Pelvic pain felt in right groin and left thigh.

Q1 Describe the X-ray appearances.

Q2 What underlying diagnosis should be considered?

Case 18

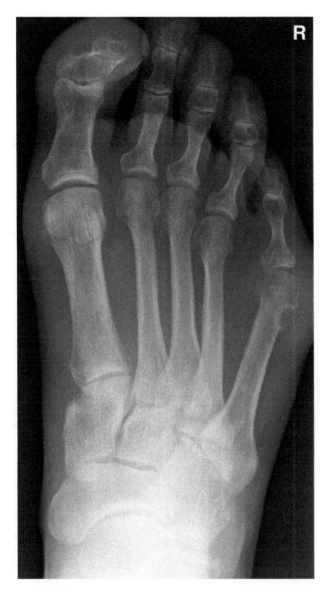

Mr FG. Age 51. Recurrent episodes of pain, redness, warmth and swelling of the right foot.

Q1 Describe the X-ray appearances.

Q2 What is the likely diagnosis?

Q3 How would you confirm the diagnosis?

Self-assessment answers

Case 1

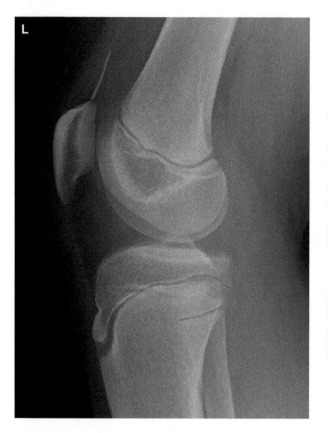

This is a lateral X-ray of the left knee of Mr A.B.

A1 The appearances are normal. At this age, the lucent lines running across the distal femur, proximal tibia and fibula are growth plates (orange). The tibial growth plate extends down to the tibial tuberosity anteriorly where it often has a wider appearance. The growth plates have smooth, undulating, sclerotic margins which would not be seen with a recent fracture.

A2 The suprapatellar pouch (yellow), outlined by darker fat planes on its anterior and posterior margins, has a normal thickness and therefore no joint swelling has been shown.

Case 2

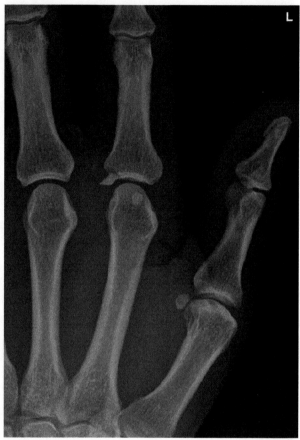

This is a magnified area from an X-ray of the left hand of Mr C.D.

A1 There is a fracture of the proximal/ulnar corner of the proximal phalanx of the index finger. The fracture involves the articular surface and the fragment has rotated approximately 45°. A second lateral view would be needed to assess displacement in other planes and look for other injuries.

A2 Obtain an orthopaedic opinion regarding reduction and internal fixation.

Case 3 (a and b)

(a)

(b)

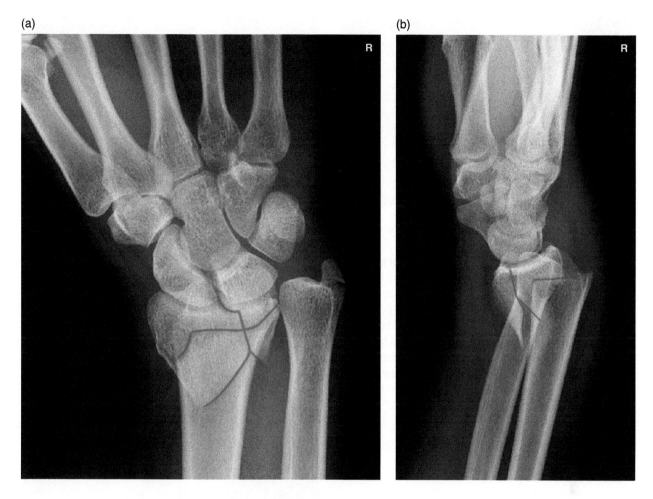

These are PA (or DP, dorsal–palmar) and lateral views of the right wrist of Ms E.F.

A1 There is an oblique fracture of the distal radius with a further sagittal fracture line extending from this to the distal articular surface. There is also a transverse fracture of the ulna styloid.

A2 The PA view shows radial shortening of approximately 1 cm. The lateral shows moderate volar (or anterior) angulation. There is no displacement where the fracture line extends into the articular surface of the radius. The ulna styloid fracture is minimally displaced.

Case 4

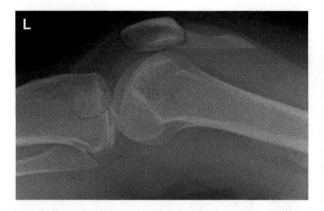

This is a horizontal-beam lateral X-ray of the left knee of Mrs S.T.

A1 There is a lipohaemarthrosis visible in the suprapatellar pouch and therefore an intra-articular fracture must be present. The top layer (yellow) is of lower X-ray density than the rest of the fluid in the suprapatellar pouch and therefore must be fat. Invariably this will have entered the joint from the bone marrow via a fracture. The remainder of the fluid (orange) will be blood due to bleeding from the fracture. A subtle fracture of the tibial plateau is visible (blue). This extends into the articular surface.

A2 An AP view.

Case 5

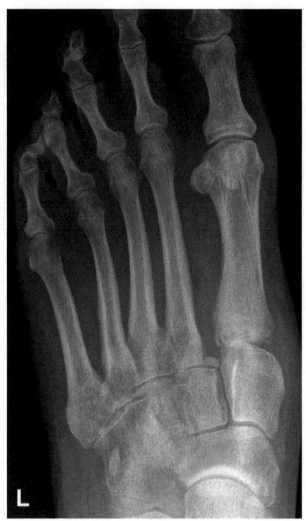

This is the straight dorsal–plantar view of the left foot of Mr G.H.

A1 There is a step visible on the medial aspect of the joint between the index metatarsal and intermediate cuneiform (follow orange line). The metatarsal is subluxed laterally by approximately 3 mm. A small bony fragment is projected over this area (yellow). The appearances are of a Lisfranc injury.

A2 An oblique view would also be needed to assess the alignment of the lateral three tarsometatarsal joints.

Case 6

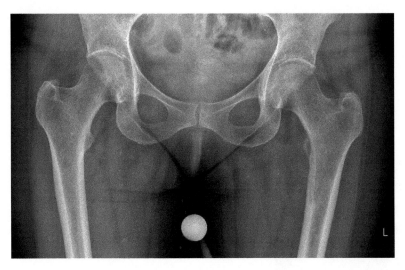

This an AP view of the pelvis and proximal femurs of Ms I.J.

A1 The medial cortex of the proximal shaft of the left femur has an ill-defined appearance (green). There is also subtle lucency of the adjacent medullary cavity and the lesser trochanter (purple). The abnormality has a wide zone of transition and is destroying the cortex, which are signs of an aggressive lesion.

A2 In this age group and in view of the previous medical history, the most likely diagnosis is a metastasis.

A3 A lateral view and X-rays of the remainder of the femur can provide useful information on the extent of the lesion and look for further distal lesions, as prophylactic nailing to prevent pathological fracture would usually be considered. MRI may also be performed to define the full extent of this lesion and show any other deposits not visible on X-ray. A radioisotope bone scan would show metastases elsewhere in the skeleton if this is required to guide overall treatment.

Case 7

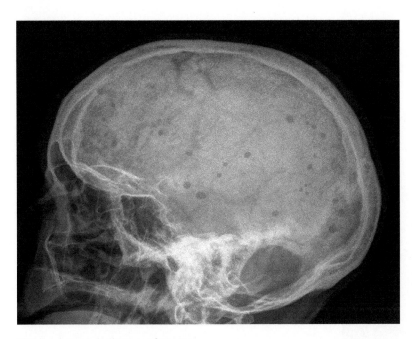

This is a lateral skull X-ray of Mr K.L.

A1 It is part of a skeletal survey to help evaluate the extent of bone changes in a patient who has been diagnosed with multiple myeloma.

A2 There are multiple, small, 'punched-out' lucent lesions scattered throughout the skull vault and a larger lucent lesion in the occipital region. The appearances are typical of multiple myeloma.

A3 An isotope bone scan would not be helpful as it does not reliably demonstrate myeloma deposits. However, an MRI of the spine may be used to show lesions not visible on X-ray.

Case 8

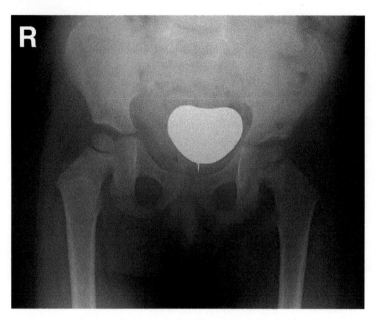

This is an AP X-ray of the pelvis and hips of Master Q.R.

A1 The most important diagnosis to consider from the clinical features is septic arthritis of the hip or osteomyelitis in the pelvis or proximal femur.

A2 There is a small area of lucency in the metaphysis of the left proximal femur. Given the clinical picture and site, this is likely to represent bone lysis from osteomyelitis.

A3 MRI would show the extent of the abnormality plus any other lesions. It will also determine whether there is any intraosseous or soft tissue abscess.

Case 9

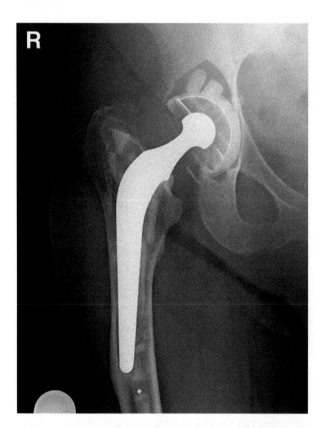

This is an AP X-ray of the right hip of Mr M.N.

A1 There is a total hip replacement. The cement around the femoral component is fragmented (orange), and there is extensive lucency surrounding the femoral and acetabular components, indicating osteolysis (blue).

A2 The appearances indicate loosening. (It is not possible to tell if the loosening is aseptic or due to infection from X-rays.)

Case 10

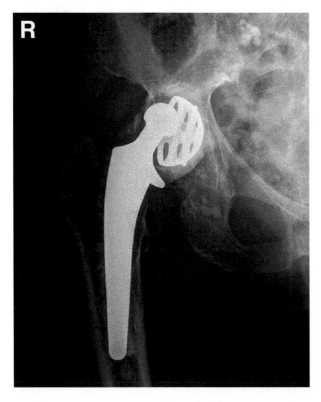

This is an AP X-ray of the right hip of Mr O.P.

A1 There is a total hip replacement. The acetabular component is rotated and no longer aligns normally with the femoral head. There is lucency between the cement of the inferior half of the acetabular component and the bone. The femoral component appears satisfactory, and there is no periprosthetic fracture shown.

A2 In view of the X-ray appearances and the clinical history, it is likely that the acetabular component is loose and has displaced acutely.

A3 Comparison with previous X-rays.

Case 11

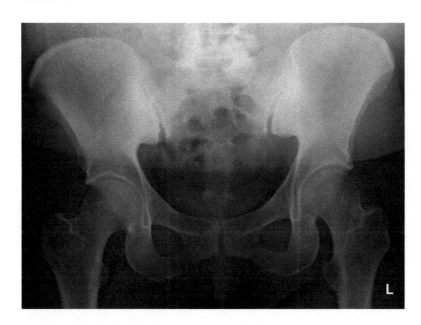

This is an AP X-ray of the pelvis.

A1 There is bilateral sacroiliitis with subchondral sclerosis (yellow) and inferior erosions (orange). Hips and entheses are normal.

A2 Axial spondyloarthritis (ankylosing spondylitis).

A3 Bony X-ray changes occur later in the disease, and MRI is much more sensitive at detecting early bone changes as well as preceding inflammation changes seen as bone marrow oedema on MRI.

Case 12

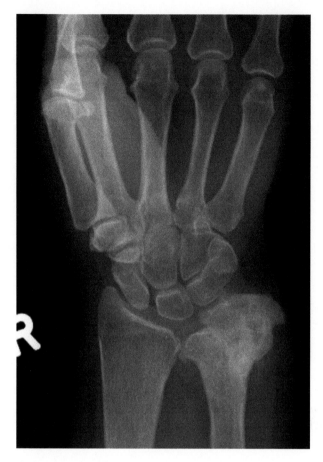

This is a PA X-ray of the right wrist.

A1 There is heavy calcification within the soft tissues surrounding the distal aspect of the right ulna bone (yellow).

A2 Calcium deposition arthropathy (probably hydroxyapatite crystals) is the likely diagnosis.

A3 Aspirate joint and examine joint fluid under polarised light microscope to look for crystals.

Case 13

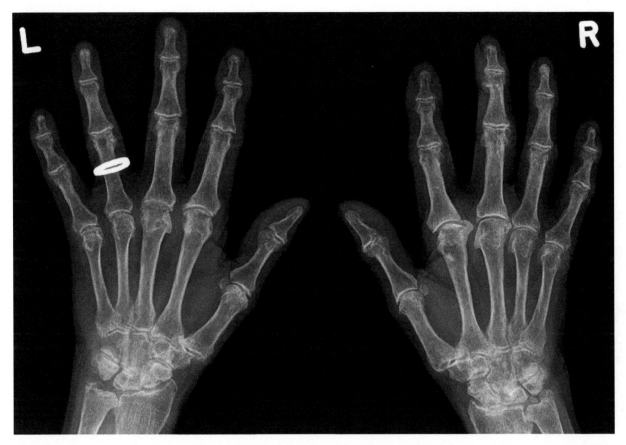

A1 This is an AP X-ray of both hands and wrists. The bones appear osteopenic. There are changes affecting thumb bases, wrists, proximal interphalangeal (PIP) and distal interphalangeal (DIP) joints with joint space narrowing and osteophyte formation. However, there is also chondrocalcinosis at both wrists (orange) and joint space narrowing (purple) with large osteophytes (yellow) particularly affecting the 2nd and 3rd metacarpophalangeal (MCP) joints, which is a more unusual site for osteoarthritis.

A2 Haemochromatosis arthropathy. Pyrophosphate arthropathy should also be considered.

A3 Serum ferritin, iron studies and genetic testing.

Case 14 (a and b)

(a)

(b)

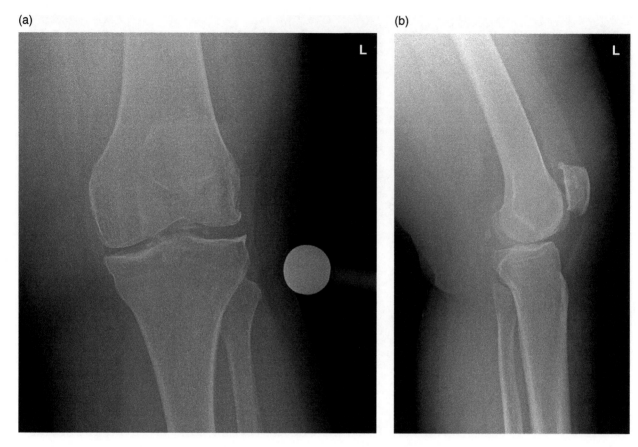

A1 These are AP and lateral X-rays of the left knee. There are changes of osteoarthritis with medial joint space narrowing (purple) and osteophyte formation (pink) and calcified bodies (blue) are visible in the suprapatellar pouch and popliteal fossa.

A2 The likely diagnosis is osteoarthritis. The calcified body may be loose but these are often adherent to the joint lining. If loose it may become stuck in the articular portion of the joint causing 'locking'. Note that the calcified body in the popliteal fossa is the fabella which is a small sesamoid bone embedded in the gastrocnemius tendon in 10–30% of the normal population. It can be seen best on the lateral X-ray but is also visible as a projection through the medial joint space on the AP image.

Case 15

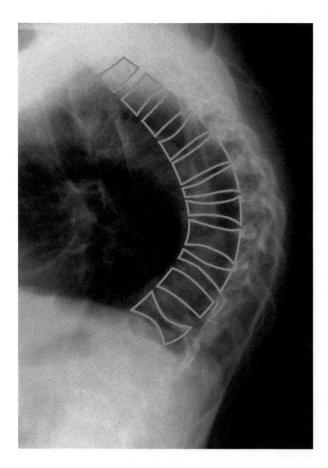

A1 This is a lateral X-ray of thoracic spine. There is a marked kyphosis with multiple thoracic vertebral crush fractures with anterior wedging.

A2 Osteoporosis.

A3 A Dual-energy X-ray absorptiometry (DEXA) scan will usually confirm a low bone mineral density, but may give a falsely high value in the presence of fractures. Note that other pathological causes of fracture cannot be excluded on plain X-rays and further imaging e.g. MRI may be required.

Case 16

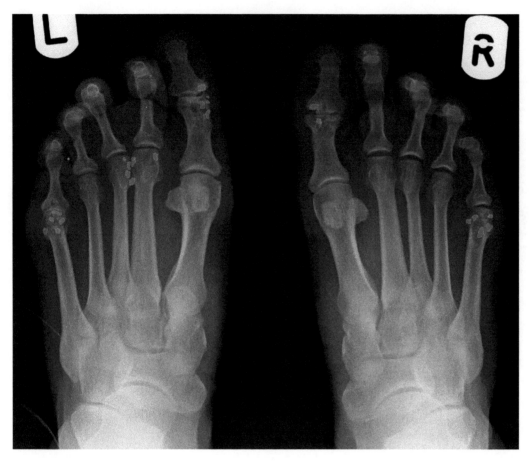

A1 This is a straight dorsiplantar view of both feet showing a symmetrical destructive erosive arthropathy (yellow) affecting symmetrical MTP and interphalangeal (IP) joints.

A2 Rheumatoid arthritis.

A3 Ultrasound or MRI.

Case 17

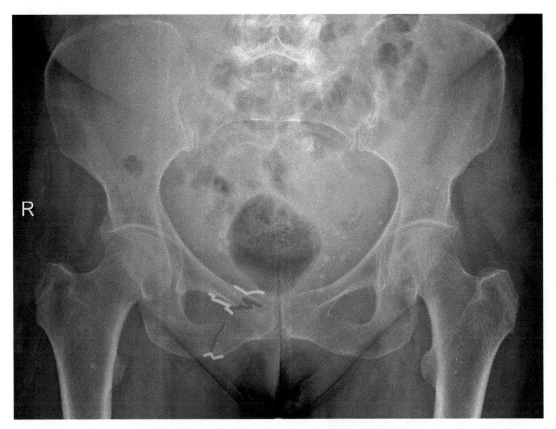

A1 This is an AP pelvis X-ray. There are fractures of the right superior and inferior pubic rami. Note the discontinuity of the bony cortex (yellow) and fracture lines (red).

A2 Osteoporosis.

Case 18

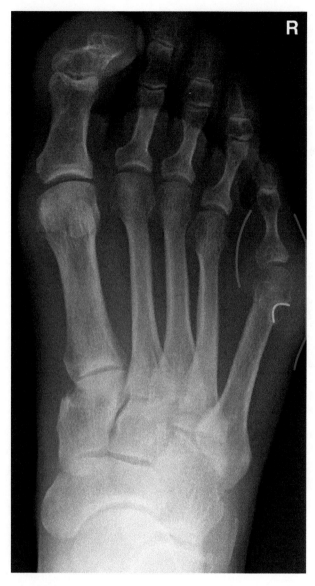

A1 This is an X-ray of the right foot. There is soft tissue swelling (orange). There is a large broad-based erosion of the lateral aspect of the 5th metatarsal neck, away from the joint (para-articular), with a 'punched out' appearance and overhanging edge (yellow).

A2 Gout.

A3 Aspirate the joint and examine joint fluid under polarised microscope to look for uric acid crystals.

Index

Musculoskeletal X-rays for Medical Students and Trainees, First Edition. Andrew K. Brown and David G. King.
© 2017 John Wiley & Sons, Ltd. Published 2017 by John Wiley & Sons, Ltd.